THYROID BALANCE

Traditional and Alternative Methods for Treating Thyroid Disorders

GLENN S. ROTHFELD, M.D., M.AC.

AND

DEBORAH S. ROMAINE

Adams Media Corporation
Avon, Massachusetts

Published by
Adams Media, an F+W Publications Company
57 Littlefield Street, Avon MA 02322. U.S.A.
www.adamsmedia.com

ISBN: 1-58062-777-3

Printed in Canada.

J I H G F E D

Library of Congress Cataloging-in-Publication Data
Rothfeld, Glenn S.
Thyroid balance / by Glenn S. Rothfeld and Deborah S. Romaine.
p.   cm.
Includes bibliographical references.
ISBN 1-58062-777-3
1. Thyroid gland—Diseases—Popular works.
[DNLM: 1. Thyroid Hormones—metabolism—Popular Works. 2. Thyroid
Diseases—therapy—Popular Works. 3. Thyroid Gland—physiology—Popular
Works. WK 202 R846t 2002] I. Romaine, Deborah S. II. Title.
RC655 .R684 2002
616.4'4—dc21
2002011332

Many of the designations used by manufacturers and sellers to distinguish their products are claimed as trademarks. Where those designations have appeared in this book
and Adams Media was aware of a trademark claim, the designations have been printed
in initial capital letters.

This publication is designed to provide accurate and authoritative information with
regard to the subject matter covered. It is sold with the understanding that the publisher
is not engaged in rendering professional medical advice. If assistance is required, the
services of a competent professional person should be sought.

This book is available at quantity discounts for bulk purchases.
For information, call 1-800-872-5627.

Contents

PART 3
Thyroid Therapies

PART 4
Restoring Thyroid Health: Living in Balance

Appendices

Introduction

You could be coming to this book for a variety of reasons. You might have a long-standing thyroid condition, and you want to make sure that you're still receiving the most appropriate treatment. You might be recently diagnosed with thyroid imbalance, either hypothyroidism (underactive thyroid) or hyperthyroidism (overactive thyroid). You might suspect that you have a thyroid imbalance but haven't gone to the doctor yet. Or you might be searching, with your doctor, to identify the reasons for your symptoms—from chronic tiredness to inability to become pregnant—and thyroid imbalance has come up as a possibility. This book is for each one of you.

READERS WITH LONG-STANDING THYROID IMBALANCE

If you've lived with underactive thyroid for years or even decades, you've no doubt adjusted to the routine of taking a pill every morning to supply your system with the thyroid hormone it needs. (The course of medication to treat overactive thyroid is limited to two years or less, so we're just addressing hypothyroidism for now.) You probably feel fine, although sometimes it's hard for you to tell because you've felt this way for so long.

And despite changes in treatment approaches and the thyroid hormone replacement drugs that are now available, you're probably still following the same treatment plan your doctor implemented when you were first diagnosed.

This is partly because you seem to be doing fine, which fits into the category of "If it's not broken, don't fix it." And it's partly because many doctors remain uninformed about new directions in thyroid treatment and are still firmly rooted in the world of "Once you start on this brand, never change." Although there is some clinical value in both of these mindsets (which we discuss throughout the book), they are just as outdated as the premise that too much sugar causes diabetes (it does not; more on diabetes and its possible relationship to thyroid imbalance in Chapters 2, 9, and 17).

When was your last checkup? What blood tests did your doctor run? How much time did your doctor spend examining your neck and thyroid gland, and talking with you about how you feel? All too often, your routine follow-up for thyroid gets minimal attention. You might even get scheduled for a brief appointment rather than a full appointment, on the premise that if you were having any problems you would've scheduled a visit specifically to address your concerns. Some doctors don't even feel the need to see long-standing thyroid patients every year! They order blood tests. If the results are within normal ranges they authorize continuing prescription refills. If the results are borderline, they'll adjust your dose and have you repeat the tests. This is not an approach that's in your best interest, even if it is expedient.

If you have a long-standing thyroid imbalance, you might not know that you're having symptoms of inappropriate thyroid hormone replacement, taking either too much or too little. And because you've been receiving treatment for so long, you probably don't think that any symptoms you do have could be connected to your thyroid. After all, *that's* under control . . . it must be something else! But your body's functions change over time, which you notice in other ways. Your thyroid function changes, too—even when you're taking medication to regulate it.

NEWLY DIAGNOSED READERS

If you're newly diagnosed with thyroid imbalance, you're probably wondering what lies ahead. If you have overactive thyroid (hyperthyroidism), your course of treatment will come to an end within a defined time, depending on which treatment option you choose (more about hyperthyroidism and its treatments in Chapters 7, 11, 17, and 18). For half of you, this will be the end of thyroid imbalance and your body will return to normal function. For the other half of you, the chapters in this book about underactive thyroid (hypothyroidism) will also become important. About half of the time, treatment for hyperthyroidism causes hypothyroidism.

When you are newly diagnosed, you have many questions that seem not to have answers. It's not really that there are no answers, but that the answers vary depending on numerous factors. This is frustrating both for doctors and for patients. Doctors like to give patients definitive information just as much as patients want to have it. But, as you'll learn as you read this book, it's nearly impossible to give a definitive answer when it comes to thyroid balance. Indeed, that's a key factor in managing thyroid balance.

As frustrating as it might be for you, treatment for underactive thyroid when you're first starting out is a matter of trial and error. Your doctor will start with a prescription for thyroid hormone replacement that he or she believes is most likely to restore optimal thyroid function. If this sounds qualified, it is. It is, at best, an educated guess! As you'll read in this book, thyroid function is a unique and moving target. What is "normal" for one person is not necessarily normal for you—not in lab results, and not in thyroid hormone supplement doses.

Doctors, like most people, have their favorite tried-and-true approaches to common problems. Thyroid disease, which currently is diagnosed in more than thirteen million Americans, is one of the most common health problems in the world. Treatment stayed the same for nearly four decades—through two and possibly three generations of doctors. With few options, doctors quickly settle into patterns of treatment—and so do you.

Research over the past five to ten years has provided a wealth of information about thyroid function, information that has not yet filtered into the general consciousness of the medical community. This new knowledge is very exciting, because it gives us insights into functions that we've so far only been able to speculate about—the role of genes in thyroid imbalance, for example, and the interrelationships between thyroid function and other endocrine function. Your doctor might be one who rides the wave of knowledge ahead of the curve of current thinking, and knows the latest findings in both the processes and treatments of thyroid dysfunction. If so, great! If not, then it's up to you to push the curve by learning as much as you can.

As someone newly diagnosed with thyroid imbalance, you find yourself scrambling to zoom from ground zero to comprehensive understanding like a dragster roars from green light to 200 mph. The difference is that the dragster has everything it needs to reach peak level in a short time, while you have to find, read, and sort through information. It can be a daunting task. Yet the only way you can collaborate with your doctor to plan your treatment approach is to have as much knowledge as possible. But unless you anticipated that thyroid balance was the problem and you've been doing a lot of reading while waiting for your lab tests and doctor's visit, your diagnosis probably caught you by surprise.

It's never too late to change, though. Starting out on one particular approach doesn't lock you into that approach. When something about your treatment seems inconsistent with what you read or hear, explore it further. If, after more extensive digging and research, the inconsistency remains, schedule an appointment with your doctor to discuss your concerns. Ask for a full-length visit, so you get enough time with your doctor.

READERS WHO ARE SEARCHING FOR ANSWERS

Perhaps you have symptoms of thyroid imbalance but either haven't gone to the doctor about it yet, or have gone to the doctor but your examination and all of your tests seem "normal." If you haven't seen your doctor yet and you have symptoms of either overactive or underactive thyroid, please schedule an appointment immediately. Although millions of people live normal, medically uneventful lives *with* treatment, going *without* treatment could cost you your health and, in rare cases, your life. These are medical conditions with potentially serious consequences if left untreated. (Chapter 14 discusses the consequences of untreated thyroid imbalance.)

If you have symptoms of thyroid imbalance but everything seems "normal," you might be feeling a little nuts right now. You might get that heavy sigh from the receptionist when you call to schedule an appointment *again*. The nurse knows you by your first name and asks about your cat. And the doctor doesn't even ask what's wrong—he just reaches to feel your neck *again*. Despite the hints, you're not a hypochondriac!

Thyroid symptoms are vague. Lab measures are becoming more precise, but there are still numerous variables that affect the consistency and interpretation of results. This makes thyroid function difficult to assess and thyroid dysfunction difficult to diagnose—particularly if you appear to be "normal." It becomes your major challenge to find a doctor who believes that your symptoms are legitimate.

This not only distracts you from focusing on your health, but also delays improvements you might feel as a result of treatment.

A number of doctors are now opting to begin treatment with a small dose of thyroid hormone replacement even when lab values and other objective measures come back normal. If you feel better as a result, does this mean you do have thyroid imbalance? It could. There's considerable debate among doctors about whether lab tests are conclusive evidence of thyroid imbalance (whether normal or not). Some doctors believe that if the lab results are normal, then the problem must be something else—even if taking thyroid hormone supplement makes you feel better. (This implies, of course, that "feeling better" is all in your head.)

If you're still searching for answers to your symptoms, keep searching. But talk with your doctor about a trial of treatment. You don't have anything to lose . . . and you have your health and peace of mind to reclaim.

AN INTEGRATED APPROACH TO THYROID BALANCE

For decades, doctors have followed pretty much the same pattern for diagnosing and treating thyroid imbalance. Identify the problem, implement the solution. We are only starting to look at health care holistically—that is, as an integration of body, mind, and spirit. Yet all of these components comprise who you are, and all of them influence your health and wellness.

ALLOPATHIC MEDICINE

Allopathic medicine is the official term for the kind of health care most Americans (and other Westerners) receive. This is the world of technology, surgery, prescription drugs, and hospitals. Doctors who practice allopathic medicine are M.D.s (medical doctor) or D.O.s (doctor of osteopathy). They study at medical schools, pass stringent exams to get licenses, and go into practice seeing patients. They follow standardized diagnosis and treatment protocols, and view health care as a process of fixing what goes wrong. This is the orientation from which your doctor functions when she says your T4 is low and prescribes thyroid hormone supplement to bring it up.

ALTERNATIVE MEDICINE

In the United States, we tend to view everything that doesn't fit the model of allopathic medicine as alternative. Sometimes we call these other approaches complementary, although a more appropriate label might be "natural." These are the traditions of health and health care that have survived in other parts of the world for centuries, such as traditional Chinese medicine (TCM), which is the foundation for therapies such as herbal remedies and acupuncture. Other alternative approaches include naturopathy and homeopathy, both of which use natural substances to interact with the human body to produce healing and protect against illness.

Although such natural systems provided remedies for thyroid imbalance long before the drugs that we use now came along, these remedies are not effective by themselves for treating either overactive or underactive thyroid. When they were the best that was available, they offered the best solution possible. Today, allopathic medicine offers more effective options and remains the recommended focal point for thyroid treatment. Many alternative approaches work well to complement and supplement allopathic treatment for thyroid imbalance, however.

INTEGRATIVE MEDICINE

Integrative medicine pulls the best from both worlds, so to speak. It incorporates the allopathic standards of diagnosis and treatment with the natural rebalancing actions of complementary or alternative approaches. If you have underactive thyroid, you need to take thyroid hormone supplement to replace the hormone your body no longer produces. This hormone is essential for the health and well-being of your entire body and all of its systems, not just your thyroid.

But if you have underactive thyroid, you have an imbalance that affects your entire body and all of its systems—physiological as well as emotional and spiritual. Approaches that restore balance to your being as a whole restore your sense of well-being. Using these methods in conjunction with conventional or allopathic approaches accommodates the infinite and intricate interrelationships that comprise your existence, not just the function of this system and that system.

ABOUT DR. ROTHFELD

Dr. Rothfeld became interested in complementary methods while studying at the State University of New York at Buffalo School of Medicine, where he received his medical degree in 1975. Upon graduating, Dr. Rothfeld worked with acupuncturists and other alternative providers, and received his first acupuncture treatment in 1979. He went on to study acupuncture himself at the Traditional Acupuncture Institute in Columbia, Maryland, and subsequently integrated acupuncture into his regular medical practice. He was astonished at the differences in how patients responded to conventional treatment in tandem with complementary methods compared to conventional treatment alone. He took a sabbatical from his practice to further his studies in acupuncture, attending the College of Traditional Chinese Acupuncture in Royal Leamington Spa, Warwickshire, England. He also received training in nutritional medicine and herbal medicine. In 1990, Dr. Rothfeld received one of the nation's first master's degrees in acupuncture. He subsequently became board-certified in the new medical specialty of medical acupuncture.

Today Dr. Rothfeld is the founder and medical director of Whole Health New England, an integrative health care practice with offices in Arlington and Plymouth, Massachusetts. There, he heads a team of clinicians in a practice that includes nutritional counseling, botanical and Chinese herbal medicine, acupuncture, natural and innovative approaches to a variety of medical problems, as well as conventional medical treatments. Dr. Rothfeld is trained in family medicine, and is a Clinical Assistant Professor of family medicine and community health at Tufts University School of Medicine in Boston. He lectures frequently. *Thyroid Balance* is his eighth book. Dr. Rothfeld's Web site, *www.thyroidbalance.com,* provides information about thyroid health from an integrative standpoint.

It is the Oath of Maimonides, a twelfth-century physician and philosopher, that inspires Dr. Rothfeld: "Inspire me with love for my art and for thy creatures. In the sufferer let me see only the human being."

Part 1

The Thyroid Butterfly: Delicate and Elusive

1

Why You Feel the Way You Do

We all have days when we wake up feeling like all we want to do is roll over and go back to sleep. When this happens once in a while, it's normal. When it happens more often than not, you certainly don't feel normal anymore. Even when you drag yourself out of bed, you lack the energy to do anything beyond what is absolutely necessary—and sometimes not even that. You forget what you set out to do, or what others tell you. You feel like confusion wraps your brain, and your thoughts seem always a half-step off. Your body aches, your hands and feet are cold all the time, and every time you see yourself in the mirror it looks like you've put on weight. Clearly something is out of balance. But what?

In all likelihood, your thyroid—and as a result, just about everything else in your body and your life.

YOUR BODY'S THERMOSTAT

Your thyroid gland perches like an open-winged butterfly across your throat, right at your Adam's apple. But don't let this gentle image fool you. This soft, delicate structure is a powerful influence on just about every function within your body. Like an organic thermostat, your thyroid gland regulates your metabolism—the collective chemical processes that run your body. When the thermostat is set too low, metabolism slows. And when it is too high, metabolism increases. Your pituitary gland, a pea-sized bundle of tissue located deep within your brain, sends the chemical signals that turn this thermostat—your thyroid gland—up and down. When these signals get confused somehow (usually when your thyroid gland responds inappropriately to them), the chemical messages that your thyroid sends out to the rest of your body also get confused. Your thyroid is then out of balance—and so is your body.

The chemical messengers in this process are hormones. There are three key hormones involved in thyroid function, although other hormones have at least minimal roles in maintaining thyroid balance (Chapter 2 gives all the details about this). Your pituitary gland releases thyroid-stimulating hormone—TSH—as the signal to your thyroid gland to produce and release its hormones. These are triiodothyronine, better known as T3, and thyroxine, or T4. Too much of these hormones signals an overactive thyroid; too little indicates an underactive thyroid. The cycle of hormone balance and imbalance is actually far more complex than this simplistic overview, of course, and we'll discuss it extensively in coming chapters.

A MATTER OF BALANCE

You hear and read a lot about thyroid *disease* or thyroid *disorders* or thyroid *conditions*. From a clinical perspective, this viewpoint is certainly valid. When thyroid function is "off," your health suffers. But so does, quite literally, every aspect of your life. More accurately, it's a matter of balance or imbalance that starts with your thyroid gland and involves every part and function of your body, from your hair to your toes. Although restoring thyroid hormone levels to "normal" levels helps to restore your body's balance, it isn't the sole solution. Balance is seldom about a single factor, but rather is a matter of how multiple factors come together to contribute to this balance. It's important to address each of these factors, as we will in this book.

Doctors typically prescribe a thyroid supplement—a drug that boosts the thyroid hormones in your system—to treat most thyroid imbalance. This is a tried-and-true therapy that has been the standard for more than a century. The earliest documented use of this therapy dates to 1891, when doctors started using ground thyroid gland tissue from sheep to treat severe hypothyroidism. In 1914, a researcher at the Mayo Clinic in Rochester, New York, isolated thyroxine, the pure extract of thyroid hormone that is still the basis of treatment today. And this therapy is an essential element in restoring thyroid balance and preventing the very serious and even life-threatening health consequences of inadequate thyroid function. (In fact, many people with hypothyroidism, or underactive thyroid, don't get enough thyroid supplementation. We'll talk more about this in later chapters.) But just as a single factor is seldom the cause of a thyroid imbalance, such a single minded approach to restoring the balance of thyroid function is often not quite enough to get you back to feeling like your normal self. Nearly everyone with thyroid imbalance feels better when they take a comprehensive, integrated approach to restoring balance to their thyroid functions, to their bodies, and to their lives. More than thirteen million Americans currently receive medical treatment to treat thyroid imbalance, and health experts estimate that as many as eight million others live with undetected thyroid problems. But simply receiving medical treatment often isn't enough to get you back to feeling normal. Countless people who are taking a thyroid supplement still suffer from subtle but disruptive symptoms such as inability to lose weight, weight gain, lack of energy, irritability and moodiness, fertility problems in women and men, and, for women, menstrual problems including premenstrual syndrome (PMS), cramping, and heavy flow. While it's bad enough to have these symptoms, what can make matters even worse is a doctor who says, "Your lab results are normal, so I don't know why you're having these problems." Lab results are important clinical measures, but they present just a piece of the picture! Unfortunately, it's the piece most doctors are trained to focus on—and if it's not the piece that fits your situation, you can find yourself hanging.

Hang no more! We know more about thyroid balance and imbalance today than we knew ten or twenty years ago when your doctor was learning about thyroid function. We know that the subtle interrelationships among thyroid hormones and other hormones in your body are just as important as the levels of thyroid hormones. We know that as many as a third to a half of all those who have underactive thyroid function have what doctors call "subclinical disease"—they don't fit the typical model when it comes to the blood tests we use to measure thyroid function. We know your blood test results can be "normal," yet you can still have the symptoms of thyroid imbalance—and we know that these symptoms can improve with a comprehensive approach that looks at your whole body as an integrated structure. We know that the way you feel is not all in your head. And we know that even people who feel fine with just thyroid supplement therapy find that they feel even better when they take a more lifestyle-oriented approach to maintaining not only thyroid balance but also body balance. From what you eat and how active you are to complementary therapies such as acupuncture and yoga, there are many factors that affect your health and well-being.

WHEN YOUR THYROID IS UNDERACTIVE

If your thyroid gland doesn't produce enough T3 and T4, the major thyroid hormones, to shut off the TSH signals from the pituitary gland, then it is underactive. This results in a clinical diagnosis of hypothyroidism, the most common thyroid imbalance (affecting about 90 percent of those who receive treatment). The classic signs of underactive thyroid include coarse hair and skin, constipation, slow but steady weight gain, feeling cold all the time, and having no energy (more about hypothyroidism in Chapter 6). Hypothyroidism tends to develop over a long period of time, often years, and becomes more common as you get older. Nearly 20 percent of women and 10 percent of men over age 60 have underactive thyroid function, although the symptoms are often attributed to other causes such as menopause or simply "aging." Although hypothyroidism is the most common thyroid imbalance, it's also the most commonly missed diagnosis, especially when the results of blood tests come back borderline or even normal.

WHEN YOUR THYROID IS OVERACTIVE

Most people with thyroid imbalances have underactive thyroid function. But your thyroid gland can kick into overdrive, too, pumping more thyroid hormones into your bloodstream than your body needs. Rather than feeling sluggish and slow, you feel all revved up. You seem to have boundless energy, and might even feel jittery. Sleep? Who needs sleep? You're hot no matter what the temperature. Your clothes seem to get looser and looser. Your heart feels like it's racing, and you might even have palpitations—those rather frightening rapid heartbeats that come one right on top of the other and make you feel like your heart is coming right out of your chest. These are the signs of hyperthyroidism, which we discuss in Chapter 7. Although hyperthyroidism is less common than hypothyroidism, it is by no means rare. Among the thirteen million Americans being treated for thyroid problems, about one million of them have hyperthyroidism. Many hyperthyroid people go on to become hypothyroid later in life, as the thyroid gland "burns out." Because hyperthyroid symptoms are more frightening and come on more suddenly, people who have them are more inclined to get to the doctor right away. And the clinical picture is clearer—just about always, the lab-test results support the symptoms.

THYROID IMBALANCE IS NOT ALWAYS A CLEAR CLINICAL PICTURE

One challenge for patients and physicians alike is that thyroid imbalances are not always clear-cut from a clinical perspective. It's dismayingly common to have a convincing constellation of symptoms that point to hypothyroidism and yet find that all the lab tests come back with results that are within normal limits. Some doctors will treat for hypothyroidism anyway, monitoring thyroid hormone levels and watching for improvements in symptoms. If you have such a doctor, give thanks! Unfortunately, the majority of doctors (especially family practitioners) just don't know enough about the subtleties of thyroid function and dys- function. Because over-supplementing thyroid hormones can cause a different set of potentially dangerous problems, many doctors who are less informed about thyroid imbalance take a "wait and see" approach, typically requesting that you return in three or six months for repeat lab tests. At best, this approach leaves you feeling as bad as ever. Or your doctor might feel com- pelled to run other tests to check for conditions such as fibromyalgia. And at worst, you might begin to wonder if maybe you're going crazy. Don't worry, you're not . . . your problems are more likely to be in your throat than in your head.

COULD YOU HAVE A THYROID IMBALANCE?

As many as eight million Americans live with undiagnosed thyroid imbalance, typically underactive thyroid. Perhaps as many who are already receiving medical treatment for thyroid imbalance continue to have symptoms. This affects your life in innumerable ways. The answers to these questions can help you determine whether you could be among them.

Questions 1–5 explore autoimmune disorders. Some forms of thyroid imbalance are the result of an autoimmune response; in other words, your body starts to view your thyroid gland as an intruder and musters an immune response to attack it. Many autoimmune disorders seem to run in families. If you or any immediate family members have an autoimmune disorder such as lupus or rheumatoid arthritis, you're more likely to develop another one such as an autoimmune form of thyroid dysfunction.

1. Does anyone in your family have a thyroid condition?
2. Do you, or does anyone in your family, have diabetes?
3. Do you, or does anyone in your family, have rheumatoid arthritis?
4. Do you, or does anyone in your family, have lupus?
5. Do you, or does anyone in your family, have pernicious anemia?

Questions 6–13 focus on problems related to dry skin and hair, common symptoms of underactive thyroid. These problems alone are not clear signs of thyroid imbalance; many things can cause dryness, from weather conditions to the hair- and skin-care products that you use. But when present with other symptoms, coarse hair and dry skin (and skin problems in general) raise suspicion about thyroid imbalance.

6. Do you frequently have dry eyes?
7. Does your mouth frequently feel dry?
8. Is your skin rough, coarse, itchy, or flaky?
9. Do you have eczema or similar skin problems?
10. Do you have vitiligo (patches of depigmented skin)?

11. Is your hair rough or coarse?
12. Do you seem to be losing hair?
13. Is your hair prematurely gray?

People with underactive thyroid typically lack energy and feel tired, fatigued, or lethargic. Questions 14–17 look at how this might play out in your life. If you feel that all you want to do is sleep and that you just don't have the energy to make it through your day, underactive thyroid could be the reason. Conversely, people with hyperactive thyroid often have trouble falling asleep or staying asleep, and feel that they have too much energy.

14. Do you have trouble falling asleep or staying asleep at night?
15. Do you have trouble waking up in the morning?
16. Do you feel that you have the energy you need to make it through your daily activities?
17. What is the first thing you want to do when you get home from work, school, or other activities?

What you eat and how your system responds, questions 18–20, are often subtle cues to your thyroid balance. Bowel movements that occur less frequently than every two or three days typically signal constipation, a sign of hypothyroidism. Bowel movements that occur several times a day, on the other hand, might signal hyperthyroidism. Cruciferous vegetables can suppress the levels of thyroid hormone in your bloodstream. Vitamin C and the B vitamins also affect thyroid hormone levels.

18. How frequently do you have bowel movements?
19. Do you eat a lot of cruciferous vegetables (like broccoli, cauliflower, cabbage, kale)?
20. Do you take vitamin supplements?

Because thyroid balance affects your metabolism, a thyroid imbalance often throws your body's heat mechanisms out of kilter. An underactive thyroid fails to maintain a high enough metabolism to generate heat to keep you feeling warm, while an overactive thyroid revs up your body's chemical processes to the point of generating too much heat. People with hypothyroidism are often cold, and people with hyperthyroidism tend to be hot. Questions 21–24 look at how your body regulates your temperature.

21. Are you frequently cold compared to other people in the same environment?
22. Are your hands and feet often cold?
23. Are you frequently hot compared to other people in the same environment?
24. Do you often have "hot flashes" in which you break out into a sudden sweat (not as a result of exercise or activity)?

Mood swings, irritability, depression, and problems with thought processes and memory (questions 25–28) are often connected to underactive thyroid. Some doctors are now looking closely at thyroid function when considering whether to prescribe antidepressants.

25. Do you easily become irritable or angry, or cry?
26. Do you feel that you have, or do others tell you that you have, mood swings?
27. Do you frequently feel "stressed out," unhappy, "down," depressed, or disinterested in life in general?
28. Are you taking any antidepressant medications?

Weight gain and loss are closely tied to metabolism (questions 29–30). If you find your weight goes up or down but you've made no changes in what you eat or how active you are, this could signal thyroid imbalance. It can also indicate other, potentially more serious, problems, so always have your doctor evaluate weight change that seems rapid and unintended.

29. Do you seem to gain or lose weight even though your eating habits have not changed?
30. Do you have trouble gaining or losing weight when you try to?

Questions 31–32 reflect the physical discomforts that plague many people who have underactive thyroid. Because these symptoms are often vague and nonspecific, it's often difficult to connect them to a specific cause until other connections fall into place.

31. Do you have a lot of body aches and discomforts?
32. Do you have fibromyalgia or a related condition?

Concentration and memory difficulties (questions 33–34) can be subtle but frustrating consequences of underactive thyroid.

33. Do you have trouble concentrating?
34. Do you frequently forget what people tell you, what you were going to do, or what you were supposed to do?

Being a woman raises the likelihood that you have a thyroid imbalance; at least 10 percent of women have underactive thyroid by the time they are 50 years old. Because the signs and symptoms of this tend to show up at about the same time menopause arrives, women and their doctors might overlook the possible connection to thyroid balance. Thyroid imbalance during pregnancy is common, and often becomes thyroid imbalance later in life. And thyroid imbalance often interferes with fertility. Questions 35–38 look at these connections.

35. Are you a woman?
36. Are you a woman of childbearing age who is having difficulty getting pregnant?
37. Are you now, or were you in the past year, pregnant?
38. Are you over age 50?

An overactive thyroid makes you feel "hyper" and jittery, and might even make you think you're having heart problems. Swelling around your thyroid gland often suggests a goiter, a swelling of the thyroid gland itself (questions 39–40).

39. Do you frequently feel nervous or agitated, and/or have heart palpitations (feel that your heart is fluttering or pounding in your chest)?
40. Does your neck look swollen, or do you have a goiter?

No single answer points the finger directly at thyroid imbalance. Collectively, however, your answers might well indicate that thyroid imbalance is a probability. Certain signs and symptoms form constellations of suspicion. If you have more "yes" than "no" answers, consider scheduling an appointment with your regular health care provider for a thyroid evaluation.

RESTORING AND MAINTAINING YOUR THYROID BALANCE

Your thyroid balance affects all aspects of your health, and, as a result, all dimensions of your life. Learning all you can about how your thyroid functions is the first and most important step you can take toward restoring and maintaining your thyroid balance. Then you can form a strong relationship with your doctor that guides you to optimal health and to feeling your best.

2

The Metabolic Matrix of Your Endocrine System

Your thyroid gland produces the hormones that regulate or play a role in nearly every bodily function—from basic growth and metabolism to the intricate hormonal balances of female fertility. It is one of the eight major structures that make up your body's endocrine system. Traditionally, doctors have thought of these structures and their functions in a fairly linear or cyclical fashion, one linked to the other. The actions of one affect the actions and reactions of others. We now know, however, that these interactions are more complex and intricate than a series of chain reactions. A shift of balance in one endocrine structure alters the balance of all endocrine structures—and of your body as a whole. The entwinement of the endocrine structures and their functions is more of a *matrix* than a linear or even cyclical relationship.

THE MOTHER OF HORMONAL ACTIVITY

The word "matrix" comes from the Latin "mater," meaning mother. A matrix is both a relationship and an environment. It supports a vast network of interactions, some of which occur in sequence and some of which take place simultaneously—and all of which are more intricately synchronized than any orchestra performance. Endocrine means "internal secretion," and this is what your endocrine structures do: They make and release biochemical substances—hormones—directly into your bloodstream. These hormones have specific and targeted missions, and their functions in your body are as precisely programmed as might be a general's battlefield strategy.

Your body's endocrine matrix extends beyond what we've traditionally viewed as the glands that comprise the endocrine system. Some organs in your body also produce hormones. Your brain itself produces endorphins and enkephalins, which act on certain nerve endings to interrupt pain signals. Your intestines secrete gastrin, secretin, and cholecystokinin, hormones that regulate certain digestive enzymes. And your kidneys produce renin, which regulates your blood pressure, and erythropoietin, which stimulates your bone marrow to make new red blood cells (erythrocytes).

All hormones come into contact with virtually all cells in your body. But a cell must have receptors for the hormone in order for the hormone to have any effect. Hormones "plug in" to these receptors, completing the circuit and initiating particular functions. For example, your pancreas produces the hormone insulin. Insulin regulates the level of glucose, or sugar, in your blood. When blood glucose levels rise, such as after eating, your pancreas releases more insulin. The insulin binds with insulin receptors in your cells, much as a key fits into a lock. The cell then "opens" to let in more sugar, which then fires up short-term energy production. Other hormones have different actions. Parathyroid hormone, which your parathyroid glands secrete, regulates the amount of calcium in your blood and bones. Melatonin, from your pineal gland, regulates your sleep cycle.

Many hormones direct other endocrine structures to produce and release their hormones, setting in motion the many cycles of function that operate your body. All of the hormones your hypothalamus produces act only on your pituitary gland, signaling it to make and release its hormones. These hormones in turn direct your body's other endocrine structures to secrete their hormones. It is an intricate and constantly shifting balance that relies on the interrelationships of numerous communication and feedback mechanisms.

Your Endocrine Glands			
Gland	**Location in Body**	**Hormones**	**Actions**
Hypothalamus	Beneath the thalamus in the center of the brain	Antidiuretic hormone (ADH)	Regulates fluid reabsorption in the kidneys
		Corticotropin-releasing hormone (CRH)	Directs pituitary to release ACTH
		Thyrotropin-releasing hormone (TRH)	Directs pituitary to release TSH
		Gonadotropin-releasing hormone (GnRH)	Directs pituitary to release FSH and LH
		Oxytocin	Contracts uterus during labor
Pituitary	Just below the hypothalamus deep within the brain	Growth hormone (GH)	Regulates growth until adulthood; strengthens muscles in adulthood; raises blood sugar levels

Your Endocrine Glands			
Gland	**Location in Body**	**Hormones**	**Actions**
Pituitary *(continued)*		Adrenocorticotro-pic hormone (ACTH)	Directs adrenals to release cortisol
		Thyroid-stimulating hormone (TSH)	Directs thyroid to release T3 and T4
		Follicle-stimu-lating hormone (FSH)	Directs ovaries to produce eggs in women; directs testes to produce sperm in men
		Luteinizing hormone (LH)	Controls egg maturation and release in women; directs testes to release testos-terone in men
		Melanocyte-stimulating hormone (MSH)	Directs skin cells to darken pigment
		Prolactin	Directs breasts to produce milk during and after pregnancy
Adrenal	One on top of each kidney	Epinephrine	Raises blood pressure, heart rate, and blood sugar level in "fight or flight" reaction
		Norepinephrine	Raises blood pressure

Your Endocrine Glands			
Gland	**Location in Body**	**Hormones**	**Actions**
Adrenal *(continued)*		Cortisol (hydrocortisone)	Maintains blood pressure; aids metabolism; reduces inflammation
		Aldosterone	Regulates sodium withdrawal by kidneys
		Dehydroepiandrosterone (DHEA)	Acts as a reserve for other hormones; cushions against stress
Thyroid	A pair of lobes across the front of the larynx	Thyroxine (T4)	Directs cellular metabolism (long-acting)
		Triiodothyronine (T3)	Directs cellular metabolism (short-acting)
Parathyroid	Two on each lobe of the thyroid gland	Parathyroid hormone (PTH)	Regulates calcium and phosphate levels
Pancreas	Behind the stomach in the upper abdomen	Insulin	Allows cells to use glucose; maintains blood glucose balance
		Glucagon	Increases blood sugar levels in response to the body's demands for energy

Your Endocrine Glands			
Gland	**Location in Body**	**Hormones**	**Actions**
Pineal	Just above the brainstem deep within the brain	Melatonin	Regulates sleep cycle
Thymus	Midchest in child- hood; vestigial in adulthood	Thymosin	Directs immune system develop- ment through adolescence
Ovaries (women)	Within the pelvic cavity in the lower abdomen	Estrogen	Directs female sex characteris- tics; regulates fer- tility cycle; readies uterus for fertilized egg to implant
		Progesterone	Directs blood vessel growth in uterus to prepare for pregnancy
		Testosterone	Affects sex drive
Testes (men)	Suspended in the scrotum, outside the body at the base of the penis	Testosterone	Directs male sex characteristics; causes sperm to mature
		Inhibin	Regulates sperm production
Placenta (preg- nant women)	Within the uterus during pregnancy	Numerous	Regulate pregnancy

COMMAND CENTRAL: YOUR HYPOTHALAMUS

The hypothalamus is actually a part of your brain rather than a distinct gland structure. It is so named because it extends from the underside of the part of your brain called the thalamus, and "hypo" means "under." Many, many nerves connect your thalamus and hypothalamus to each other so that even though they are two structures, they are physically inseparable. Through a complex combination of nerve signals and chemical messages, your hypothalamus manages key functions essential for life, such as those that regulate breathing, heart rate, and blood pressure. The hypothalamus also maintains your body's fluid balance and body temperature, and produces the hormones that direct the activities of all the other glands in the endocrine system. This is why the hypothalamus is called "command central."

The hormones your hypothalamus produces include:

- Antidiuretic hormone (ADH), which regulates fluid reabsorption in the kidneys to maintain appropriate fluid levels in your body
- Corticotropin-releasing hormone (CRH), which directs the pituitary to release ACTH
- Thyrotropin-releasing hormone (TRH), which directs the pituitary to release TSH
- Gonadotropin-releasing hormone (GnRH), which directs the pituitary to release FSH and LH
- Oxytocin, which causes the uterus to contract during labor, and is involved in the sexual response

The thalamus is the portion of your brainstem that enters your brain. It functions as a switchboard of sorts, linking your unconscious and conscious nervous-system functions. Your hypothalamus is an extension of this filtering and transmittal function. Your hypothalamus receives nerve and chemical signals—the feedback mechanisms—from the thalamus, and directs actions within your body that address the needs these signals reflect.

Say, for example, that you drop a book on your foot. Your thalamus receives the nerve impulses that race from your foot up your nervous system and spine and into your brain. Some of the signals pass through to other parts of your brain, which then directs actions such as causing you to clutch your foot as you hop around on the other one. These responses remove you from the danger. And some of the signals go to your hypothalamus, which instructs your adrenal glands to release epinephrine, so you're ready to flee from the cause of the injury, and cortisol, to soothe the inflamed tissues where the book hit your foot.

Your hypothalamus also initiates thyroid action. When your hypothalamus receives the message that the circulating levels of thyroid hormones are too low, it sends a jolt of thyrotropin-releasing hormone (TRH) to your pituitary gland. Your pituitary, in turn, releases thyroid-stimulating hormone (TSH), which signals your thyroid gland to release its hormones. Once the message comes through the thalamus to your hypothalamus that thyroid hormone levels in your blood are adequate, your hypothalamus shuts off the TRH, your pituitary shuts down its production of TSH, and your thyroid stops releasing its hormones.

It is very rare that a problem with your hypothalamus causes thyroid imbalance. Most hypothalamus problems result from bleeding that affects the area (such as from severe head trauma or a stroke) or from tumors involving the surrounding tissues (like the pituitary).

SERGEANT AT ARMS: YOUR PITUITARY GLAND

Your pituitary joins to your hypothalamus along a short bundle of nerve tissue, suspended just below it. It receives its marching orders from your hypothalamus, and then directs the other endocrine glands to make appropriate responses and actions. Like a sergeant at arms, your pituitary gland maintains order within your endocrine matrix. It also produces some of your body's most important hormones. Although it is no larger than a pea, the pituitary gland has three clearly distinct lobes: anterior, mid-pituitary, and posterior. Each produces certain hormones.

The anterior lobe is the most active. It produces:

- Growth hormone (GH), which regulates growth until adulthood, strengthens muscles in adulthood, and raises blood sugar levels
- Adrenocorticotropic hormone (ACTH), which directs the adrenal glands to release cortisol
- Thyroid-stimulating hormone (TSH), which directs the thyroid gland to produce and to release its hormones
- Follicle-stimulating hormone (FSH), which directs the ovaries to produce eggs in women, and the testes to produce sperm in men
- Luteinizing hormone (LH), which controls egg maturation and release in women (the menstrual cycle), and directs the testes to release testosterone in men

The pituitary's other two lobes have limited and specialized functions. The mid-pituitary produces melanocyte-stimulating hormone (MSH), which directs the skin cells to darken pigment. The posterior lobe produces prolactin, which directs the breasts to produce milk during pregnancy and lactation (while a woman is breastfeeding).

When your pituitary gland receives TRH from your hypothalamus, it releases thyroid-stimulating hormone (TSH). This directs your thyroid gland to release its hormones. When your hypothalamus gets the message that your thyroid hormone levels are adequate, via various biochemical signals that reach it through the endocrine matrix as well as the neurotransmitter network, it turns off the TRH. As the TRH level drops off, your pituitary stops secreting TSH. This in turn causes your thyroid to stop releasing thyroid hormones.

For decades doctors have believed that thyroid function was a fairly self-contained stimulation-response cycle. New research shows us that in fact these cycles are complex interrelationships that link with each other in multiple ways. TSH not only promotes the production as well as the release of the thyroid hormones, but also controls their conversion in the liver and tissues (more about this in Chapter 3). This is an important extension in our understanding of the thyroid gland's role.

Although rare, tumors are the primary cause of problems with the pituitary gland. Pituitary tumors can affect any of the gland's hormonal functions. A tumor that causes a decrease in TSH results in underactive thyroid; one that causes TSH secretion to increase causes overactive thyroid. If, for any reason, it would be necessary to remove your pituitary gland (such as to treat a tumor), you would become permanently hypothyroid. You then would need to take thyroid supplements and carefully monitor your thyroid functions for the rest of your life. However, pituitary-related thyroid problems are extremely uncommon.

SWEET DREAMS: YOUR PINEAL GLAND

On the other side of your brainstem, tucked away at the back edge of where the cerebrum meets the cerebellum, is the somewhat mysterious pineal gland. The pineal's conical shape and reddish color give this gland its name, which means "pinecone-like." Because of its location deep in the center of the brain, the pineal gland was called the "third eye" by ancient physicians. The pineal gland has just one known function: it secretes melatonin, a hormone that appears to regulate the sleep cycle.

There is still much that we don't know about melatonin,

but that knowledge is increasing as is the field of chronobiology, the study of biology in relationship to time. Melatonin is produced during darkness from serotonin, a brain neurotransmitter that is critical for mood and well-being. Melatonin is related to your body's circadian cycle—the coordination of your rhythm of sleeping and waking to the cycles of light and darkness. Because sleep refreshes us, it makes sense that the hormone that the body produces mainly when we sleep is involved in regenerating activity. Melatonin appears to be necessary for a healthy immune system, for good blood sugar balance, for proper menstrual cycles, and, of course, for a restful sleep. Although clearly there is some connection to metabolism, since metabolic functions ordinarily decrease during sleep, as yet there is little research to confirm this. We do know that melatonin levels rise significantly during hibernation in animals such as bears. At the same time, body temperature drops and metabolism slows, but we don't know enough about how or why this is the case to be able to link melatonin and metabolism conclusively.

THE THERMOSTAT: YOUR THYROID GLAND

Your thyroid gland stretches across the front of your neck, its two lobes straddling your larynx. A thin band of tissue, called the isthmus, links the two lobes. This unassuming gland looks like a pinkish lump of spongelike material. Under a microscope, this material appears as tiny sacs clustered together like bunches of grapes. Your thyroid gland produces two key thyroid hormones, thyroxine, better known as T4, and triiodothyronine, or T3. Other thyroid hormones that are derived from T4 and T3 are reverse T3 (rT3) and diiolo-L-thryonine, or T2. Chapter 3 discusses these hormones and their functions.

Your thyroid also secretes the hormone calcitonin, which regulates the balance of calcium in your bloodstream and in your bones. When calcitonin levels go up, calcium leaves your bones and enters your bloodstream. When calcitonin levels go down, calcium leaves your blood and goes into your bone tissue. In this manner, there is an inverse relationship between calcitonin and parathyroid hormone, which also affects blood and bone calcium levels. However, there doesn't seem to be a direct relationship between calcitonin and the thyroid hormones.

Thyroid promotes growth hormone production, which promotes growth in infants and children and has a role in healthy aging of adults. Lack of thyroid hormones in a developing child (before as well as following birth) often causes irreversible damage to the brain that results in intellectual impairment. Most hospitals routinely test the blood of newborns for thyroid hormone levels. Underactive thyroid is a frequent cause of fertility problems. And thyroid imbalance contributes to unhealthy aging.

BONE BALANCE: YOUR PARATHYROID GLANDS

These four tiny glands dangle in two pairs from the tissues of your thyroid gland, although they are not actually part of the thyroid. "Para" means "around." Your parathyroids produce parathyroid hormone, which regulates the balance of calcium and phosphate in your body. This balance is essential for strong, healthy bones, and also for proper heart function (calcium plays a key role in transmitting the electrical impulses that cause your heart to beat). The relationship between your thyroid gland and your parathyroids is in fact one based on the respective roles the glands play in maintaining your body's calcium balance rather than on their physical proximity to each other. Problems that affect the parathyroid glands can influence your thyroid gland's calcitonin feedback mechanism, resulting in levels that are too high or too low.

If you've had your thyroid gland surgically removed, your parathyroid glands go, too. You can maintain your body's calcium balance by taking supplements containing calcium and other nutrients that promote bone growth (more on this in Chapter 15). Proper hormonal balance, good quality sleep, and stress reduction also have profound effects on bone health, since stress will increase the body's cortisol, leading to loss of bone. Dietary factors also are critical, both in getting enough dietary calcium and also avoiding foods that leach calcium from bones, such as sugar and carbonated soft drinks (particularly colas).

FIGHT OR FLIGHT: YOUR ADRENAL GLANDS

Not only do you have a pair of adrenal glands, resting like caps over the tops of your kidneys, but your adrenal glands also are really two organs in one. The adrenal medulla, the inner portion of the adrenal gland, is, like your hypothalamus, intimately connected to your nervous system. It produces the neurotransmitters (sometimes called neurohormones) epinephrine and norepinephrine, which govern your "fight-or-flight" response. Epinephrine and norepinephrine jolt key functions into high gear, most notably breathing, heart rate, and blood pressure. The adrenal medulla receives signals directly through your nervous system as well as through the secretions of your pituitary gland.

The adrenal cortex, the outer layer of the adrenal gland, secretes several hormones that have both maintenance and stress response functions. These hormones include:

- Aldosterone, which controls how much sodium your kidneys pull out of your bloodstream to maintain blood volume and pressure
- Cortisol, or hydrocortisone, which controls how your body metabolizes and uses fats, proteins, and carbohydrates as well as playing a role in your body's anti-inflammatory and recovery responses

- Dehydroepiandrosterone (DHEA), which acts like a reserve to both the adrenal and sex hormones. This steroid hormone can be converted into testosterone or progesterone, or used as raw material to produce cortisol in times of stress.

Your adrenal glands release their hormones when your pituitary's release of ACTH signals them to do so. There is growing evidence that there is a subtle but significant interrelationship between adrenal function and thyroid balance (more about this in Chapter 8).

GENDER-SPECIFIC GLANDS: TESTES AND OVARIES

The glands that determine your sex characteristics—ovaries in women and testes in men—produce what are probably the most noticeable endocrine effects. These glands give you your physical definition as male or female and establish fertility. In women, the ovaries produce estrogen, progesterone, and small amounts of testosterone. Estrogen and progesterone levels rise and fall as a woman's menstrual cycle unfolds. These hormones also take on expanded roles during pregnancy, first supporting and then encouraging the conclusion of the unborn baby's stay in the uterus. In men, the testes produce testosterone, commonly known as the "male hormone," and another hormone called inhibin, which regulates how sperm develop.

Thyroid hormones are crucial to proper functioning of the reproductive systems in both men and women. Underactive thyroid in women can suppress ovulation and make the menstrual flow unusually heavy. It also affects emotional ups and downs related to fluctuating progesterone levels, making PMS more severe. Overactive thyroid in women also can suppress ovulation, but lightens or even stops the menstrual flow. Either imbalance affects fertility as well as a woman's sense of well-being.

In men, thyroid imbalance affects sperm production and maturation, with either underactive or overactive thyroid causing a drop in sperm count and motility that results in decreased fertility. A severely underactive thyroid during adolescence can interfere with growth and development, causing slow physical maturation and delays in secondary sex characteristics.

We now know that male and female sex hormones have roles in both sexes. In women, testosterone promotes a healthy sexual response (libido), enhances lubrication of vaginal tissues during sex, and helps build bone density. In men, small amounts of estrogen and progesterone may be important in protecting the prostate gland from too much testosterone stimulation.

THE DYNAMICS OF BALANCE

The new understanding about the endocrine matrix that is emerging from recent research is changing our entire perspective on thyroid balance and imbalance. Although present medical approaches to treatment, such as hormone supplements or replacements, remain valid and important, we are learning that every change made to one part of the matrix affects all of the other parts. And sometimes, what we perceive as a problem in one part is actually a reflection of problems somewhere else in the matrix. For some people, restoring thyroid balance might always be as simple as a pill a day. For a growing number of others, however, the dynamics of balance extend well beyond the thyroid.

3

Thyroid Function and Dysfunction

The word "thyroid" comes from two Greek words, "thyreos" and "eidos," that mean "in the form of a shield." And it is like a shield that your thyroid gland spreads across the front of your trachea. It's an appropriate image for what we are now learning is the surprising role that the thyroid gland has in protecting your body from the stresses of living. Does this warriorlike image startle you? It might well! The traditional view of the thyroid gland has been that it is quite delicate and mysterious, likened to the equally delicate image of a butterfly. Visually, this image remains appropriate. But as modern technology reveals the deepest secrets of the activities and functions of cells, the minutiae of cellular communication and interaction, it is becoming clear that this complex gland is but one dimension of a metabolic matrix that links the multitude of hormones—the biochemical messengers—that give your body its marching orders.

THYROID CHEMISTRY 101

Your thyroid gland produces two key thyroid hormones, thyroxine, better known as T4, and triiodothyronine, better known as T3. The cells in your thyroid gland make these hormones from two substances that come from your diet, the element iodine and the amino acid tyrosine. T4 is so nicknamed because it contains four iodine atoms, and T3 because it contains three iodine atoms. The ebb and flow of TSH that your pituitary releases determines the ratio of bound to free T3 and T4, which remains relatively constant when your thyroid is in balance. Your thyroid stores these hormones within its cells, and then secretes them in response to TSH from your pituitary gland.

Converting T4 to T3

The majority of thyroid hormone in your system, about 80 percent, is T4, but most of the thyroid hormone that enters your cells is T3. T3 and T4 are present in your bloodstream in two forms, bound and free. Bound T3 and T4 are attached to proteins, which keeps them from having any action on cells, and are in plentiful supply. The supply of free T3 and free T4, the forms these hormones must be in to have an effect on your cells, is very limited—only about 1 percent of T4 and 5 percent of T3 are free. As your cells draw in free T3 and free T4, however, bound T3 and T4 break away to become free, replacing what the cells use.

T4 is very slow-acting, and T3 is very fast-acting. Your body needs both forms to function properly. T4's effect is slow and long-acting, covering days, while T3 hits fast and then is gone. T4 also is a storage form of thyroid hormone that your body converts, by removing an iodine atom, into the active form T3. Cells in your liver and certain other body tissues make this conversion. The resulting thyroglobulin molecule takes one of two forms. The active form is T3, and the inactive form is called reverse T3 or rT3. Like so many systems in the body that have two hormones or systems that balance each other, T3 and rT3 have opposite effects. T3 speeds up metabolism, and rT3 slows it down. This becomes especially important when we look at the effects of stress on metabolism, as we will in Chapter 8.

THYROID HORMONES AND CELL METABOLISM

T3 and T4 play essential roles in cell metabolism. Your cells require two kinds of fuel, glucose (sugar) and oxygen. Insulin regulates how cells use glucose, and thyroid hormones regulate how cells use oxygen. When a T3 or T4 molecule enters a cell, it must "plug in" or bind to a thyroid receptor in the cell. This "opens" the cell to receive oxygen molecules. The cell "burns" the oxygen, which creates chemical interactions that release energy and heat to fuel your body's functions.

The energy the cell generates through this sequence of events goes outward, to meet the needs of other cellular processes. The cell needs its own supply of energy so it can make this energy. So your pancreas sends insulin, which binds with the cell's insulin receptors. The cell opens itself to accept glucose, which it then burns to fuel its own needs. All of these interactions then cause you to feel hungry, your body's signal that you need to replenish its supply of the raw materials it uses to create the fuels it feeds your cells.

NEW LEARNING: DIVING INTO
THE DEEP END OF THE GENE POOL

We've known since the 1970s that thyroid hormones link to receptors within cells. These receptors determine the level of thyroid hormone that enters the cell. Thanks to genetics research conducted in the 1990s, we now know that there are two specific genes that determine how these receptors receive thyroid hormone. It's very likely that these genes are responsible for how effectively thyroid supplements function when given to treat hypothyroidism as well. We anticipate that as we learn more about the gene link and how it affects thyroid receptiveness, we will gain insight into why conventional treatment relieves symptoms for some people with underactive thyroid but not for others.

We also know that many variables influence the genetic response accountable for thyroid function, including environment (such as iodine or radiation exposure) and nutrition (including hormone-producing vitamins such as retinoic acid and vitamin D). We'll come back to these factors in later chapters. It is possible, though as yet unproven, that there is a genetic connection to underactive thyroid, with changes in the genes (mutations) setting the stage for disruption in the thyroid cycle and perhaps in the endocrine matrix as a whole.

CHARTING NEW TERRITORY

Many of our new understandings come from one of the most ambitious scientific research projects of all time, the Human Genome Project (HGP). Initiated in 1990, the HGP set out to identify, or map, the entire sequence of genetic information that defines the human being. Ever since British scientists James Watson and Francis Crick gave us the familiar spiral staircase representation of DNA (deoxyribonucleic acid) in 1953, the molecule that contains genetic information, researchers have worked to unravel the mysteries of the body's functions.

Researchers completed the preliminary gene sequence in 2001, identifying and locating the 35,000 genes that form the basis of instruction for human existence. The findings promise to completely change the way we think about how the human body functions, in health (balance) and disease (imbalance). We've long suspected that genetic instruction is responsible for both function and dysfunction; now we have evidence. When genetic instructions become distorted, they alter the functions they direct.

The mapping of the human genome—the blueprint of the human body—is showing us glimpses of its complex and elegant system of genes and chromosomes, a system that defines every detail of the body's form and function. No longer do we think of genes as volumes in a library containing the history of our formation. We now know that physiology is not the independent functioning of discrete systems within the body. Rather, it is a dynamic amalgam of cells, tissues, hormones, and tissue-based messengers and sensors, all of which constantly receive and give information and readjust responses to affect the whole body. Your body is, as we talked about in Chapter 2, a network of complex and interrelated functions that form an intricate matrix of parts and functions.

WHERE THE ACTION IS: THE SECRET WORLD OF MITOCHONDRIA

We've known for thirty years now that thyroid action is a function of molecular biology, not just a matter of chemistry. That is, it takes place at the level of molecules and as a function of living mechanisms. What we haven't known until recently is precisely how those functions take place, because they happen deep within elements of the cell, which have been just beyond the reach of technology. But now new technologies have allowed researchers to "drill down" to new layers of understanding about how metabolism functions inside the cell, at the mitochondrial level.

Mitochondria are the smallest units of biological function within the cell, and each cell contains hundreds and sometimes several thousand of them. Each mitochondrion has its own DNA, providing detailed instructions for the intricate and focused functions it carries out. It is the mitochondria that actually perform the tasks of living, on a submicroscopic level. At the end stage of metabolism, mitochondria create the energy your body needs. They do this by combining molecules of oxygen with molecules of other substances such as amino acids and sugars to create a chemical "fuel" called adenosine triphosphate (ATP). Mitochondria also manufacture certain steroid hormones (such as testosterone) and elements of cell DNA.

When a thyroid hormone molecule binds to a thyroid receptor in the cell, it must also bind to certain DNA structures on specific genes within the mitochondria. Mitochondrial function governs this binding, determining how much binding takes place. This, in turn, affects how much the thyroid hormone can stimulate cell activity and influence metabolism. And here's where the new insights gained through the Human Genome Project and other genetic research become significant. It appears that another form of thyroid hormone, diiolo-L-thryonine, or T2, similarly binds to receptors within the mitochondria. (We have to say "appears" because as yet researchers have not been able to directly observe this mitochondrial binding, but what they can observe leaves little doubt that this is what happens.)

The implications of this discovery are exciting and far-reaching. While we have known of T2's existence for quite some time, we have viewed it not as an active form of thyroid hormone but rather as a by-product of some sort, resulting from the removal of yet another iodine atom, presumably as T3 was used, and then expelled by the cells. And we have known that underactive thyroid causes slowed metabolism (accounting for symptoms such as fatigue and lethargy).

These new findings show us how and why. The process of converting T4 to T3 is amazingly complex and intricate, and only part of the picture. T2 is not inactive, as we have long assumed, but in fact might be the most significant form of thyroid hormone in your body. The thyroid influence penetrates to the very core of cellular function, to mitochondrial activity. This helps to shape the genetic directives that mitochondria give to cells, which might explain the autoimmune aspect of thyroid imbalance. And it directly affects the amount of energy (in the form ATP) that mitochondria produce.

As our understanding of mitochondrial function has grown, we've learned that mitochondrial dysfunction is the underlying cause of such devastating diseases as muscular dystrophy.

Disrupted mitochondrial respiration allows toxins to build up within the cell, causing cell damage and even death. This damage affects multiple body systems. This knowledge has led to new treatment approaches for mitochondrial disorders that focus on the body as a whole rather than just the disease's symptoms. When we apply our knowledge of mitochondrial function and dysfunction to thyroid imbalance, particularly underactive thyroid, the seemingly diverse and disconnected range of symptoms begins to make more sense.

- *High blood cholesterol:* One function of mitochondria is to break down fatty acids. When this function becomes impaired, fatty acids accumulate in your blood. Decreased thyroid activity can raise blood lipids (such as cholesterol), since thyroid hormone is necessary to break down LDL cholesterol. LDL is what we think of as "bad" cholesterol; it is thick and sticky, and clings to the insides of the walls of your arteries. Eventually this results in narrowing and blockages, leading to an interruption of blood flow that can cause a heart attack or a stroke.
- *Fatigue and lethargy:* Problems in converting T4 to T3 to T2 directly and indirectly affect mitochondrial energy production. The energy that does get produced goes first to your body's high utilizers, your vital organs—heart, lungs, brain, liver, kidneys.
- *Weight gain:* Lowered mitochondrial energy production means lower metabolism. Your body uses less of the fuel—food—that you supply to it. There is some speculation that when metabolism reaches a certain low point, your body kicks into "starvation survival mode," further slowing metabolism in an effort to conserve fuel. But the problem isn't with the fuel supply; it's with fuel use. So you keep eating to give your body fuel, but there's reduced consumption at the mitochondrial and cell levels.

- *Feeling cold:* T4 to T3 conversion plays a key role in the process through which your body activates heat-producing mechanisms. When T3 levels are low, these mechanisms fail to activate.
- *Cognition and memory difficulties:* Disrupted mitochondrial function that affects nerve cells in the brain interferes with their ability to work properly and efficiently, perhaps slowing synapses (communications across cells) as well as functions within the cells.

And of course, all of these actions and reactions affect each other as well as literally every function in your body. It's more than just a cause-and-effect relationship; not only does one action lead to another to another to another, but each of those "anothers" leads to other chains of actions and reactions.

YOUR THYROID OUT OF BALANCE

Your body is a constantly adjusting matrix of information, with everything affecting everything else. Thyroid function is part of this intricate balance. Thyroid hormones affect, and are affected by, many other hormones in the body. A thyroid out of balance affects just about every function in your body. Some effects of thyroid imbalance are so specific, however, that we look for them as part of the diagnostic journey.

METABOLISM: WHAT'S UP (OR DOWN) WITH YOUR WEIGHT?

Eons ago, our primate ancestors traveled long distances in search of food. Their bodies developed a physiological way of ensuring that they would have the energy necessary for their trek, even when calories were scarce. When limited food supplies forced them into fasting, the thyroid compensated by automatically slowing down the body's metabolism to conserve energy. Today, this feature of thyroid function has become the dreaded "set point" so critical to people trying to lose weight (which we'll discuss further in Chapter 16). Now we have foods of many lands at our fingertips, but the thyroid system that adjusts our metabolism with efficiency and promptness still functions as it did ages go.

How efficiently your body burns fuel determines its caloric needs. When your metabolism is sluggish, as happens with underactive thyroid, your body doesn't burn fuel as efficiently as it could. One result is a slow but steady weight gain. No matter how much or what you eat, no matter what your activity level, your weight keeps creeping up. You feel tired and sluggish as well, because your body's metabolism isn't generating enough energy to make you feel energized. The consequences of this can be far-reaching, as it can cause many of your body's systems to slow or even shut down. Slow metabolism is a reminder for your body that serves as a "starvation" alert. Your body perceives that it is not getting enough fuel, since it doesn't have enough energy. So it begins to conserve energy, further slowing metabolism.

The reverse situation exists with overactive thyroid. No matter how or what you eat, no matter your activity level, you keep losing weight. Your metabolism has kicked into overdrive, and your cells are merrily burning away as much fuel, in the form of oxygen, as they can acquire. Your body's feedback mechanisms interpret this as meaning that your cells need even more fuel, and your endocrine system cranks up another notch. This hypermetabolic pace is hard on every system in your body, particularly your heart. It cranks up the pace, too, beating more rapidly and harder to try to keep a steady supply of oxygen flowing to the cells that are demanding it to meet their metabolic needs.

THERMODYNAMICS: RUNNING HOT, RUNNING COLD

As your body's master gland, your hypothalamus collects a vast amount of information through various means (such as nerve impulses and chemical signals). It responds to even the most minute of changes in your body's multitude of balances faster than your brain can consciously register them, sending its own signals to make whatever adjustments are necessary. When the temperature outside your body is cold, your hypothalamus signals your pituitary gland to release TSH, which in turn signals your thyroid to kick up the thermostat a bit—in other words, to increase your metabolic rate to generate heat as a by-product of the chemical reactions of metabolism. When the temperature outside your body is hot, your pituitary gland slows or even temporarily stops releasing TSH, allowing your metabolism to slow and your internal body temperature to cool.

When your thyroid is overactive, it's stimulating your metabolism too much. The high level of chemical reactions that result means that your body is constantly generating heat—"burning" fuel. It's not just that you *feel* hot; your body temperature actually rises. This activates other responses in your body that attempt to disperse the excess heat—sweating, for example. The result is that you begin looking for ways to help your body cool down, such as throwing off the covers or shedding clothing. Conversely, when your thyroid is underactive it is not maintaining a high enough metabolic rate. There just aren't enough chemical reactions to keep the "fire" going, and your body temperature drops. This correspondingly activates other body responses that attempt to stoke the "fire" and bring the temperature up. You feel cold, pull on more blankets or put on more clothes, and might even shiver.

As your thyroid hormone imbalance becomes more pronounced (which will happen until medical treatment intervenes to start restoring balance), your body gets trapped in whichever reaction mode is appropriate. If your thyroid is overactive you sweat and feel hot all the time, and if your thyroid is underactive you just can't get warm. Because individual tolerance to heat and cold varies widely, however, and because thyroid imbalance (particularly underactivity) can take years to develop, you might accept that you're just "hot-blooded" or "cold-blooded" without considering that there could be an underlying imbalance that is the cause. Most people don't perceive simply being consistently too cold or too hot as a health matter or enough of a reason to see a doctor.

BEYOND THE SURFACE: SKIN AND HAIR

Your skin and hair are often the first outward signs of thyroid imbalance; since they are fast-growing tissues, they rapidly show the effects of abnormal metabolism. When your thyroid is underactive, your skin becomes dry and even scaly. Your hair becomes coarse and falls out easily. These are the effects of slowed metabolism and lack of nourishment reaching the outermost parts of your body. When your thyroid is overactive, you might have oily skin and hair and excessive sweating (especially your palms). Your skin becomes moist and perhaps reddened, as though you are extremely hot (which your body believes you are). These are the effects of accelerated metabolism. Although these problems are seldom serious, they can be distressing. Fortunately, they go away once your thyroid balance is restored.

MOODY AND BLUE: EMOTIONS, COGNITION, AND MEMORY

Thyroid imbalance has a clear effect on your moods and emotions, in part through its effects on your nervous system and in part because thyroid imbalance affects the many interrelationships among all of the hormones in your body. There is also evidence that the autoimmune component of hypothyroidism affects nerve and brain cells. (Chapters 6 and 7 discuss thyroid balance and its effects on the brain.) Overactive thyroid can leave you feeling edgy and irritable, while underactive thyroid often leads you to mild depression.

Certain life events—most notably pregnancy, menopause, and aging—confuse the matter of thyroid balance and brain function. Your body's needs for thyroid hormones increase during pregnancy, and it is common to develop underactive thyroid at this time. But it's also common for pregnant women to experience mood swings and even difficulties with memory and thought processes, which doctors believe result from the fluctuations of hormones, including thyroid hormones, during pregnancy. Menopause is another time in a woman's life that typically is marked by changes in emotional responses, memory, and thought processes. And mental processes tend to decline in both men and women as a common aspect of aging. This makes it difficult to determine the real reasons for these changes.

Although doctors are beginning to routinely check for thyroid imbalance, many times they don't consider the potential of underactive or overactive thyroid until other symptoms show up. By that time you might truly feel like you're losing your mind! Therapy that brings your thyroid functions back in balance ends these kinds of problems if they are in fact thyroid-related.

RESTORING THYROID BALANCE

In most situations of thyroid imbalance, restoring balance involves a combination of therapies and approaches. There is no "one size fits all" treatment; each person's thyroid balance is unique, and so are the approaches to restore balance. The vast majority of people with thyroid imbalance take thyroid hormone supplement or other medications to alter the chemistry of their bodies. Adding other approaches that fit with your lifestyle—from nutritional changes to acupuncture, chiropractic, and yoga—complete the picture. The critical point is that the thyroid gland is very sensitive to both our external and internal environments, and any approach to balancing its function needs to include attention to those environments.

4

Metamorphosis: A Good Diagnosis Can Transform Your Life

A good diagnosis often can be more elusive than the butterfly that the thyroid resembles. Experts believe that up to 40 percent of adults have some level of thyroid imbalance, primarily underactive thyroid. Some of these millions of people have no idea that the headaches, chronic tiredness, emotional ups and downs, and other discomforts that plague their daily lives might actually have physical origins. Because these are the malaises of our modern, stressful times, it's easy to write them off as inevitable consequences of lifestyles that are too hectic. Many people don't even view them as medical problems with potential medical solutions.

Others among the millions with undiagnosed thyroid imbalance have been to see more doctors than they can count, more times than they can count. And they've also gotten more "diagnoses" and treatment recommendations than they can count. Headaches? Try a pain reliever. Tired all the time? Go to bed earlier. Emotions taking you for a ride? Consider counseling and the antidepressant du jour. While each of these recommendations has merit, each is offered in isolation. That is, they don't look at the whole picture as a collection of discomforts that might, just might, have a common cause.

Even among those who do receive a diagnosis of thyroid imbalance, an unknown percentage continues to feel less than 100 percent well even after treatment, and further testing establishes that their bodies have returned to normal. Their thyroid tests might show normal levels of T3, T4, and TSH, but still they feel out of sorts. Things aren't quite what they used to be, aren't quite right, aren't what the doctors implied they would be. "You're getting older . . . you can't expect to feel twenty-five years old all of your life!" True enough. But there's no reason to expect a steady downhill slide, either!

Why is diagnosis so difficult? After all, it's easy enough to measure the thyroid hormones in your body . . . isn't it? For the majority of people with thyroid imbalance, the answer is yes. Tests that measure the levels of T3, T4, and TSH in your blood are easy to do and, when the results are abnormal, can provide conclusive clinical evidence that your thyroid function is out of balance. But blood tests aren't everything, and aren't always enough to provide a conclusive diagnosis. While they can quantify amounts, even microamounts, of myriads of chemical substances in your body, blood tests cannot measure how these substances interact with each other or with the cells that carry out the operations of your body's functions. In fact, most of the function of thyroid hormones, and most of where they malfunction, occurs within the mitochondria of cells, out of the reach of standard measurements. And medical treatment isn't the end-all, be-all, either. Despite the many marvels of its intricate design and structure, your body is not a machine. Maintaining its health is a delicate and sometimes elusive balance.

ANCIENT CHALLENGE

Thyroid imbalance is among the oldest ailments known to humankind. Skeletal remains recovered from archeological sites all around the world, dated to be thousands of years old, show evidence of the kind of bone damage typically found as a consequence of untreated thyroid imbalance. Overactive thyroid drains calcium from the bones, resulting in the kinds of fractures associated with conditions such as osteoporosis, particularly compression fractures of the spine and fractures at the wrists—places where fractures due to injury are uncommon. Underactive thyroid in young people causes bone growth to end prematurely. While other signs of aging might exist in the skeleton, telltale signs of early growth cessation, such as calcification in the area of the growth plates, remain as evidence that thyroid hormones were in short supply during critical development periods. Yet it wasn't until the twentieth century that there were effective medical treatments to correct thyroid imbalance.

By the Middle Ages, records document a problem then known as "cretinism," a condition of severe thyroid deficiency in infancy and early childhood that results in permanent brain damage, severe intellectual impairment, and stunted physical growth. (Today we call this disorder congenital hypothyroidism.) Though the term eventually took on the pejorative meaning "idiot," originally it simply meant "little Christian"—a reflection of the belief that those afflicted with such severe handicaps were the innocent children of God. This problem was especially common in the inner mountain regions of the area that is now Switzerland and the mountainous regions of what are now Spain and Italy—which we now know reflects the lack of iodine in the water supply in geographic environments far from the ocean.

In the sixteenth century, one European physician espoused a new view: the human body was a balance of chemistry. The radical views of Philippus Aureolus Theophrastus Bombast von

Hohenheim (1493–1541)—better known as Paracelsus—transformed medicine, pushing understanding of the body's functions to new levels. Also trained as an alchemist, Paracelsus combined his knowledge of chemistry as it related to metallurgy with his observations of chemistry as it related to the human body. Paracelsus was the first to document the link between cretinism and goiter, and between goiter and diet. His travels took him all over Western Europe, and led him to observe that people who had goiters were far more common in regions away from the coast, and that the children who suffered from a form of severe mental retardation known then as cretinism nearly always had mothers who had goiters. This led Paracelsus to conclude that there was something in the water.

Indeed, Paracelsus was right. Sea water contained high concentrations of iodine, while inland waters contained little if any iodine. Iodine intake, as we now know (although Paracelsus did not), is essential for the body to manufacture thyroid hormones. There are no records to prove whether Paracelsus took his conclusions to the next logical step and prescribed sea water for people with goiters, although this did later become a folk remedy for goiter.

IF WE CAN FIND IT, WE CAN FIX IT

The orientation of modern allopathic medicine—the kind of medicine your family practitioner, internist, or endocrinologist practices and that is most common in Western cultures—has become "find it and fix it." This is not a criticism; the technology that makes this orientation successful has saved untold lives and improved the quality of life for all of us. It is the orientation that has improved life for millions of people with diagnosed thyroid imbalances. But it is an orientation with limitations. The "find it and fix it" approach views the body's organs and functions in relative isolation. A heart attack, for example, is a problem that involves one organ, the heart. A kidney stone is a problem that involves a different organ, the kidney. Technology can pinpoint the problem and its damage, and help doctors "fix" the problem using, perhaps, fairly high-tech solutions such as surgery and drugs.

But the human body doesn't function in isolation. As independent as certain organs and organ systems might appear, they are nonetheless intricately interwoven with one another. A heart attack involves damage to the heart, certainly. But it reflects a cumulative shift in the body's environment—perhaps clogged arteries from excessive blood cholesterol that a high-fat diet and inactive lifestyle allow to accumulate, with high blood pressure a result. Blood surging through the arteries at increased pressure dislodges a fragment of cholesterol, or cholesterol accumulates on the insides of the arteries serving the heart to the extent that blood can no longer pass through them. Result: heart attack. Change any of these contributing factors, however, and you alter the course of the heart's health. This holistic view of heart disease has become popular over the last ten years or so, as we have earned more about the role of lifestyle in health and disease.

We are making similar strides in understanding the connections between lifestyle and thyroid imbalance, too. But these advances are not as widely known. In fact, even among those who should be in the know—physicians—information is sometimes sketchy at best. Many doctors, too many doctors, continue to evaluate and treat thyroid conditions following the same guidelines they learned in medical school ten, fifteen, twenty (or more) years ago. They rely almost exclusively on laboratory findings to determine diagnosis. And they tend to dismiss symptoms that don't fit the traditional assessment framework, either as irrelevant or as signs of some other health problem. If they can't find it (lab tests don't verify it), then they can't fix it.

In June 2000, the American Thyroid Association (ATA) acknowledged the limitations of the "find it, fix it" orientation and issued revised guidelines calling for U.S. physicians to routinely screen for thyroid function in all patients, starting at age 35 and repeating the screening every five years in the absence of symptoms. Previously, guidelines recommended only symptom-based testing. In explaining its new position on thyroid screening, the ATA said:

> Clinical manifestations of thyroid dysfunction vary consider-ably among patients in their character and severity. Associated symptoms and signs are often nonspecific and progress slowly. Consequently, the accuracy of clinical diagnosis is limited. Physicians must consider and exclude thyroid dysfunction much more often than they will establish a diagnosis. If only patients presenting with clearly suggestive symptoms and signs are evaluated, many affected individuals will remain undiag-nosed. For these persons, appropriate treatment for thyroid dysfunction or conservative monitoring to anticipate its poten-tial future consequences can only be implemented when rou-tine laboratory screening identifies them.

Even with routine screening, diagnosing thyroid imbalance remains more art than science. Many people have lab-test results that are within normal limits, yet they also have symptoms of thy-roid imbalance (particularly underactive thyroid). They often have what doctors call "subclinical disease"—while they don't have the clinical signs of dysfunction, they do have symptoms suggesting that things are not quite right. It is possible to have a thyroid imbalance and have normal lab tests. There's more to thyroid balance and imbalance than what can be measured by conventional means (as Chapter 5 discusses in detail).

FINDING THE RIGHT TREATMENT BALANCE

Nearly all thyroid imbalance involves a certain level of "find it, fix it" and will require a level of medical intervention; the challenge lies in finding the treatment approach and balance that works best for you. Many people with thyroid imbalance will find that they need to take thyroid supplements for the rest of their lives. It is essential to make sure your body has an adequate supply of thyroid hormones, and as yet there is no known way to force your thyroid gland to produce this adequate supply except through hormone supplementation. There are various products available, each with advantages and disadvantages, so you do have options and choices. Dietary and lifestyle factors are important integrative elements for everyone with thyroid imbalance, and many people benefit from complementary therapies such as acupuncture and yoga.

Your goal—and your doctor's—should be to find the right balance of methods so that you can enjoy your life to the fullest. Restoring thyroid balance often requires patience and persistence as you try various supplement products and doses, blending the medical treatment aspect with other changes and adjustments. You need to find the hormonal balance that is optimal for your body, as measured by lab tests as well as by your symptoms and how you feel. This process is the most frustrating part of thyroid imbalance. But that balance does exist!

FINDING THE RIGHT DOCTOR

Doctors who diagnose and treat thyroid imbalance include family practitioners, internists, and endocrinologists. Although there is no official specialty practice area in thyroid disorders, some doctors have special interest in thyroid function and dysfunction, and correspondingly have additional expertise and knowledge. Finding a doctor who is a good match for your interests and needs can be as much of a challenge as is restoring your thyroid balance. This is a personal as much as a medical matter. Of course you want to choose a doctor who has the qualifications to evaluate and treat your thyroid condition. You also want a doctor who sees thyroid balance in the context of your overall health.

Ask your doctor about his or her level of interest in thyroid disorders. What typical approaches does your doctor favor? "I generally use some form of thyroid supplementation combined with other approaches that help restore your health to its fullest" is a great response. "I see where the lab values are, and adjust Synthroid levels accordingly" is a response that might suggest this doctor has a rather narrow view of thyroid balance. Does your doctor use words such as "function" and "dysfunction" when talking about your thyroid, or "disease" or "disorder"? These words might reflect a traditional allopathic orientation that leaves little room for "thinking outside the box." Does your doctor talk about "balance" and "imbalance," about "lifestyle" and "quality of life"? This language demonstrates an understanding that the thyroid is but one dimension of the complex and intricate design that is your health and wellness.

FINDING THE RIGHT DIAGNOSIS

The search for your diagnosis should be as integrative as your eventual treatment, and most of the time is a multistep process that doesn't just end with a prescription. Diagnosis typically begins with a clinical assessment that includes physical examination and laboratory tests. Your doctor should take some time to feel your neck, evaluating your thyroid gland for swelling or nodules. Your doctor should order a comprehensive series of lab tests to measure your thyroid's functions, following up with other kinds of tests if appropriate, to get a complete picture of your body's hormonal and chemical balances. In some situations, your doctor might also order tests such as ultrasound, thyroid scan, or biopsy to provide further information. (Chapter 5 discusses the various tests that can help identify thyroid imbalance and problems.) And your doctor should also take time to ask you questions, and to listen to your answers. These questions should include many of those we asked in Chapter 1; your answers will establish a baseline of general wellness that reflects the overall balance of your health and also points to any thyroid imbalance.

The next step in your diagnostic journey should be a follow-up visit to discuss your test results, not just as numbers and values, but also as they might relate to your symptoms. At this visit, you and your doctor should decide together what is the most appropriate step to take next. If your lab tests come back with normal values but you still have symptoms of underactive thyroid, discuss with your doctor the possibility of beginning trial treatment with thyroid supplements to see if that improves the way you feel. "Normal" is simply a range, and not everyone fits into it. Your doctor should monitor the changes in your lab values, both to make sure your thyroid hormone levels remain safe and to find the levels at which you feel your best.

5

Traditional and Alternative Thyroid Testing Methods

Tests that measure thyroid function have been around for decades, and for decades they have shaped treatment modalities. Following this mostly linear view, doctors have treated the thyroid gland as though its functions could be measured and addressed in isolation from the rest of the body. We now know that this is shortsighted and inappropriate; the functions of your thyroid gland affect, and are affected by, many other functions in your body. Lab tests and clinical findings are but the *first* steps in looking at your thyroid balance.

The method of measuring thyroid hormones in the blood, called the radioimmunoassay (RIA), was developed in the 1970s by American physicians Solomon Berson and Rosalyn Yallow, who won the 1977 Nobel Prize in Medicine for their work. This sophisticated technology now makes it possible to measure hormone levels in the bloodstream with great precision. The most common tests measure blood levels of thyroid and other hormones, while scans and biopsies give doctors unique and often revealing looks at the inner workings of your thyroid gland.

So start your diagnostic journey with these lab tests; they give you very important information about your thyroid gland's functions. But then look at the results as snapshots that you must arrange in such a way that they present a panorama of your thyroid in the context of other metabolic and body functions. This will help you find the path, the integrative approach, to restoring balance that works best for *you*.

BASELINE BLOOD TESTS: THYROID PANEL

Most doctors start the diagnostic process by ordering blood tests collectively known as a thyroid panel to provide a baseline assessment of the levels of thyroid hormones in your bloodstream. Some doctors like to order just a TSH and Total T4 as a preliminary screening tool, mostly as a cost-saving measure to appease insurance companies that balk at paying for full testing, especially when symptoms are vague. This combination is effective only when the results are conclusive for underactive thyroid. When results are inconclusive or normal, further tests are necessary. Various factors can affect the results of these blood tests, including birth control pills, hormone replacement therapy (HRT), estrogen replacement therapy (ERT), beta-blocker medications (such as those used to treat high blood pressure), some medications for seizures, and a low-carbohydrate diet (such as with many weight loss programs).

A typical thyroid panel includes these blood tests:

- High-sensitivity thyroid-stimulating hormone assay, commonly called TSH or sTSH. This test measures the amount of thyroid-stimulating hormone in your blood, which your pituitary gland releases to signal your thyroid gland to release thyroid hormones. The higher the value, the greater the amount of TSH in your blood and the stronger of a signal that your thyroid needs to initiate its functions. A value above 2 microunits per milliliter of blood (2 mU/ml) raises the suspicion that thyroid function might be a bit sluggish; a value above 5 mU/ml is considered clinically conclusive of hypothyroidism (underactive thyroid). There is some variation of normal values among laboratories.

- Serum thyroxine, also called total thyroxine, total T4, or T4. This test measures the total amount of thyroxine, free and bound, in your blood. A low value indicates underactive thyroid, and a low T4 in combination with an elevated TSH pretty clearly points to the thyroid itself as the source of the imbalance. A low T4 with a normal or low TSH suggests that the problem lies with the pituitary gland rather than the thyroid gland. A high T4 points to overactive thyroid, although certain circumstances (like taking HRT) lead to elevated T4 without hyperthyroidism.

- Serum triiodothyronine, or total T3. This test measures the total amount of triiodothyronine, free and bound, in your blood. A high T3 indicates overactive thyroid. Because T3 is more sensitive than T4, its levels can rise much earlier than do T4 levels, so it is not uncommon to have a high T3 with a normal T4 in hyperthyroidism. A low T3 suggests hypothyroidism, although drugs such as steroids and certain blood pressure medications can cause a falsely low result.

- Resin T3, Resin T4 Uptake. When done in conjunction with a total T3 and a total T4, these tests are sometimes referred to as a T7. Performed only in conjunction with either total T3 or total T4, resin uptake helps determine whether variations in T3 or T4 are truly the result of altered thyroid function or are instead related to thyroid binding. Results that are opposite—high T3 or T4 and low resin uptake, or low T3 or T4 and high resin uptake—suggest underactive or overactive thyroid, while results that are the same—low/low or high/high—suggest that binding is the issue. Estrogens, such as are in birth control pills and HRT, can decrease thyroid binding, which causes a falsely low T3 or T4 resin uptake, with elevation of free T3 or T4.

ADDITIONAL BLOOD TESTS TO MEASURE SPECIFIC ASPECTS OF THYROID FUNCTION

Your doctor might request additional blood tests that specifically measure certain aspects of thyroid function. These tests are most useful when initial tests return inconclusive results or negative results even though you have symptoms that suggest thyroid imbalance. They include:

- Free T4 (FT4) measures the amount of free (unbound) T4 in your blood. Higher-than-normal values suggest underactive thyroid, and lower-than-normal values suggest overactive thyroid.
- Free T3 (FT3) measures the amount of free (unbound) T3 in your blood. Higher-than-normal values suggest underactive thyroid, and lower-than-normal values suggest overactive thyroid. T3 levels are more sensitive and change more quickly than T4 levels.
- Reverse T3 (rT3) measures the circulating amount of this substance, which is formed along with T3 when T4 is broken down. The rT3 level has been associated with a functionally low thyroid in the face of normal hormone levels.
- Thyroid-binding globulin (TBG) measures the amount of tyrosine-containing protein that binds to iodine to form thyroid hormones. High or low levels of TBG, which can happen in certain situations, will lead to falsely aberrant thyroid hormone levels.

- Antithyroid microsomal antibodies and antithyroglobulin antibodies often are present in Graves' disease (a form of hyperthyroidism) and Hashimoto's thyroiditis. When these antibodies are present, it indicates that there is an autoimmune process going on. However, these antibodies are present in a number of autoimmune conditions besides thyroid disorders, such as systemic lupus erythematosis (SLE) and type 1 diabetes (childhood onset). For this reason, positive antibodies don't by themselves indicate thyroid imbalance, but rather present small images of the total metabolic matrix picture.

- Anti-TPO (thyroperoxidase) antibodies, which are antibodies to a thyroid-related enzyme, are more likely to suggest thyroiditis. Again, the result of this test has to be evaluated in the context of the bigger picture. Lack of these autoantibodies does not rule out the possibility of Hashimoto's thyroiditis.

- Radioactive iodine uptake (RAIU) involves giving you a pill containing radioactive iodine (in an amount that is harmless to your health). Several hours later, a scan detects the concentration of iodine in your thyroid gland (see the section "Looking Deeper: Thyroid Ultrasound and Scans" later in this chapter). This is an important way that doctors assess whether your thyroid is overactive, taking up higher amounts of iodine than normal. In addition, the RAIU scan, or thyroid scan, will show if there is a thyroid nodule, an isolated mass of thyroid tissue that has increased (or decreased) thyroid function.

This chart summarizes the blood tests commonly performed to assess thyroid function:

Thyroid Blood Tests

Test	Measures	Normal Ranges	Below-Normal Result Suggests	Above-Normal Result Suggests
TSH or sTSH	amount of thyroid-stimulating hormone in the blood	0.5 mU/ml–5.5 mU/ml	overactive thyroid (hyperthyroidism)	underactive thyroid (hypothyroidism)
serum thyroxine or total T4	amount of thyroxine (T4) in the blood	4.6–12 ug/dl	underactive thyroid	overactive thyroid
free thyroxine or FT4	amount of free (unbound) T4 in the blood	0.7–1.9 ng/dl	underactive thyroid	overactive thyroid
serum tri-iodothyronine or total T3	amount of total T3 in the blood	80–180 ng/dl	underactive thyroid	overactive thyroid
free tri-iodothyronine or FT3	amount of free (unbound) T3 in the blood	230–619 pg/d	underactive thyroid	overactive thyroid
reverse T3 or rT3	amount of rT3 in the blood	% correlation to T3 and T4	clinical situation other than or in addition to thyroid imbalance	clinical situation other than or in addition to thyroid imbalance

Thyroid Blood Tests *(continued)*				
Test	**Measures**	**Normal Ranges**	**Below-Normal Result Suggests**	**Above-Normal Result Suggests**
thyroxine-binding globulin (TBG)	amount of tyrosine-containing protein in the blood	12–20 ug/dl T4 + 1.8 ugm	clinical situation other than or in addition to thyroid imbalance	clinical situation other than or in addition to thyroid imbalance
radioactive iodine uptake or RAUI	amount of iodine that concentrates in the thyroid gland	10–30 percent	underactive thyroid or thyroid nodule	overactive thyroid or thyroid nodule
antithyroid microsomal antibodies/ antithyroglob-ulin antibodies	antibody presence	positive or negative	inconclusive	inconclusive
anti-TPO anti-bodies	antibody presence	positive or negative	inconclusive	inconclusive

OTHER BLOOD TESTS

As we've described in earlier chapters, thyroid hormone production and release involves an intricate cycling of hormones involving not only your thyroid gland but also your hypothalamus, pituitary gland, and sometimes other glands such as your adrenal glands. It's sometimes helpful, especially if the thyroid panel returns inconclusive results, to obtain additional blood tests.

Two other tests can be performed to further identify the source of thyroid dysfunction. These tests, which are usually performed in a hospital or specialist setting because they are so complex, help determine whether thyroid imbalance is the result of pituitary imbalance:

- TRH stimulation involves giving you an injection of thyroid-releasing hormone (TRH) to stimulate your pituitary gland to release thyroid-stimulating hormone (TSH), and then measuring your serum TSH level, as a test of whether your pituitary gland is functioning properly. A low TSH (indicating a low response to TRH) may demonstrate low pituitary function, while a strong TSH response suggests that the thyroid gland is the issue.
- TSH by IRMA (thyroid-stimulating hormone measured by immunoradiometric assay) is a very sensitive test that measures the amounts of TSH as they change in response to amounts of T3 and T4 in your blood. TSH by IRMA identifies the failure of your pituitary gland to respond to dropping T3 and T4 levels, which ordinarily cause the pituitary gland to release TSH.

Of course, the thyroid does not function in isolation but exists within the metabolic matrix that controls all of your body's functions. Adrenal and liver function, sex hormones, and nutritional testing all are important to assess the proper function of this matrix.

LOOKING DEEPER:
THYROID ULTRASOUND AND SCANS

Thyroid scans give doctors the chance to look at the functions of your thyroid gland without cutting into your body.

- Ultrasound uses high-frequency sound waves to create a dimensional image of your thyroid gland. (This is the same technology that shows the developing baby inside a pregnant woman's uterus.) It is painless. Ultrasound is typically used to help evaluate nodules and lumps; it easily determines whether a nodule is a fluid-filled cyst or is a mass of solid tissue. This determination guides further diagnostic decisions.

- Radioactive iodine uptake (RAIU) scan involves having you take a pill that contains radioactive iodine. After several hours, the iodine makes its way into your bloodstream, where your thyroid "uptakes" or absorbs it. The thyroid is the only tissue in your body that absorbs iodine; making the iodine radioactive allows special cameras to take pictures of how the iodine concentrates in your thyroid gland.

  There are three kinds of RAIU scans, rectilinear, gamma camera, and computerized rectilinear. A rectilinear scan creates an image on paper of your thyroid gland, true to scale (real size). This allows doctors to measure its size and dimensions, and also to measure any nodules that are present. A gamma camera scan uses a camera sensitive to radioactivity to take a picture of your thyroid gland. The computerized rectilinear scan, developed in the 1990s, is rapidly becoming the scan of choice because it measures both appearance and function of the thyroid gland. This gives incredibly accurate analysis of thyroid balance and imbalance, and is particularly useful in monitoring treatment effectiveness for overactive thyroid (hyperthyroidism).

- Radioisotope scans include another radioactive isotope, such as technetium, with radioactive iodine to provide more refined measurements of thyroid function. These substances "light up" your thyroid gland on the scan.

Normally functioning thyroid tissue absorbs these isotopes in certain ways; thyroid tissue that is not functioning normally absorbs them in different ways and concentrations (or doesn't absorb them at all).

Despite their high-tech nature, scans by themselves don't give a complete picture of your thyroid's function. Most often, doctors order scans in conjunction with other tests (including standard and specialized blood tests) to provide additional details that help them make the correct diagnosis. Just as with blood tests, however, scan results can be normal or inconclusive—which doesn't either diagnose or rule out thyroid imbalance.

EXAMINING CELLS: BIOPSY

If there is a lump or nodule on your thyroid gland, your doctor might want to look at the cells it contains under a microscope to determine whether they are cancerous. The procedure involves inserting a thin needle into the lump and withdrawing some cells. Sometimes ultrasound is used to help guide the needle into the nodule. The needle is very fine, and the procedure is quick, safe, and generally doesn't involve any discomfort. Most (95 percent) of thyroid lumps and nodules are *not* cancer.

NONTRADITIONAL TESTS

Body temperature has always been an indicator of general health. Mostly, we watch for elevations, telling us that fever is present—a clear sign of infection. Only recently, however, have we recognized that low body temperature is also a health indicator as well as a window into the body's hormonal cycles. Women can chart their fertility cycles, for example, by plotting their daily body temperatures on a graph. Over a typical 28-day cycle, body temperatures rise and fall by as much as 2°F. Rising body temperature indicates a shift in a woman's hormonal balance that signals ovulation—her most fertile time. There is a similar, although not cyclical, correlation between body temperature and thyroid hormone levels. Dr. Broda Barnes pioneered use of basal body temperature as a diagnostic tool for underactive thyroid (although not one that has yet gained widespread acceptance among doctors with traditional views of thyroid function). Basal body temperature is particularly useful in identifying subclinical hypothyroidism—underactive thyroid with lab results that are within normal limits or just slightly askew.

This method involves taking your body temperature immediately upon waking in the morning, using an old-fashioned mercury thermometer placed under your arm for ten minutes. The Broda Barnes method has people do this every day for ten days. (Because a woman's body temperature changes over the course of her fertility cycle, a woman should take her waking basal body temperature during the week she is menstruating.) If your waking basal body temperature is consistently below 98.2°F, it's highly likely that you have underactive thyroid. Some doctors find this a more helpful indicator than blood tests, particularly when test results are inconclusive or even come back normal. And this is something you can do at home, on your own, to give you a better idea whether your symptoms reflect a sluggish metabolism that thyroid treatment might address. Hyperthyroidism, however, does not correlate with elevated temperatures, and blood tests are still considered the most diagnostic.

Another test your doctor might perform is called the Achilles tendon reflex. With you seated and your feet dangling, your doctor taps your Achilles tendon (along the back of your heel). This causes your calf muscle to contract and your foot to jerk downward. A slower-than-normal reaction suggests under-active thyroid, reflecting the slowed metabolic activity of the muscle cells as they respond to the Achilles stimulation. This test isn't necessarily conclusive, but does provide an additional clue about the state of your thyroid balance.

WHEN YOUR TEST RESULTS ARE "ABNORMAL"

Abnormal thyroid test results are considered clinically conclusive evidence of thyroid imbalance, and your doctor will want to initiate prompt treatment. It's important to restore balance to your thyroid function and to the rest of your body. The longer your body functions in a state of imbalance, the more likely it is that you'll experience continuing symptoms and that you might cause serious harm to your body. Which treatment, precisely, is used depends first on whether your thyroid appears to be underactive or overactive, and second on whether your thyroid imbalance appears to be primary (your thyroid gland itself is the source of the imbalance) or secondary (another health problem or disease is creating a thyroid imbalance). Your key challenge when your thyroid test results are abnormal is to find the balance of treatment and lifestyle that works best for you, that helps you feel like yourself again. We explore treatment options in later chapters. So are all of your problems over, now that testing has revealed a thyroid imbalance? Most of the time, abnormal test results lead to the treatment that restores not only your thyroid balance, but also your sense of well-being. It remains important to have regular blood tests to make sure your thyroid hormones stay within normal limits. It's also important for you to keep track of how you feel and whether your symptoms go away entirely or tend to go away for a while and then come back. If the latter, you probably need to fine-tune your medical treatment and take a closer look at the lifestyle factors that influence thyroid function, such as diet and activity. Remember, blood tests are just snapshots of what is going on within your body *at that moment*. In reality, your body is a web of constantly changing information, responding at each moment to the messages of your environment.

RETESTING TO KEEP UP
WITH CHANGES IN YOUR LIFE

If you become more physically active because you now feel so much better, great! You're likely to lose weight (a blessing if your thyroid imbalance has impeded your efforts to do so until now) and gain muscle mass as your physical activity level rises. If you experience greater than a 10 percent weight loss, have your doctor run another thyroid panel just to be sure that your thyroid hormones are still within normal limits and at a healthy balance. A more fit and trim body often has a higher metabolism and functions more efficiently; the dose of thyroid supplement that was appropriate when your imbalance was first diagnosed might be too high for the new and improved you.

And remember that as your life changes, your thyroid balance changes. As your body ages, your metabolic functions slow and change. Menopause and pregnancy—because of their significant hormonal shifts—are points in a woman's life at which those functions change dramatically, and because your thyroid gland is your body's metabolic thermostat, it has a clear and significant role in those changes. If you are "manually" adjusting that balance through treatment (as compared to the "automatic" adjusting your body would do if you didn't have a thyroid imbalance), you might need to adjust your thyroid supplement dose to accommodate those changes. Other factors influence this balance, too, such as soy products and herbs you might take, especially during menopause. (More about this in later chapters, as we further explore the concepts of metabolic balance throughout your body.)

Although the metabolic changes of aging are less dramatic for men, their bodies, too, undergo hormone shifts as they grow older. Metabolism slows, and it might be necessary to increase your thyroid supplement dose. Are you a man in midlife to late life who has added a lot of cruciferous vegetables and soy products to your diet to improve your prostate health or to help you fight prostate cancer? The chemicals in these foods, namely isoflavones, are powerful anticarcinogens, but they also suppress thyroid function (more on this in later chapters). This is a natural benefit if you have overactive thyroid, but not such a good thing if you have underactive thyroid. Again, regular blood tests can help you stay on top of your body's changing needs.

WHEN YOUR TEST RESULTS ARE "NORMAL"

As much as hearing your doctor say, "Everything's normal!" might bring a sigh of relief, these words also bring a sigh of frustration because they mean your quest for diagnosis continues. This is almost always a circumstance that occurs when symptoms suggest underactive thyroid. Your doctor might choose to begin treating you with thyroid supplements anyway, and monitor your blood thyroid levels over the next six months to a year to see what, if any, changes treatment produces in them as well as in how you feel. Some people feel sluggish with a TSH around 3, right in the center of "normal," while others feel a bit jittery at the same value. Always remember that normal is a range; the lab values that you have when you feel at your best are the ones that are healthy and normal for you.

Doctors who treat a lot of thyroid imbalance have come to recognize that even the most subtle shifts in lab values can result in significant differences in terms of how you feel and what symptoms you have. And we also have learned much just in the past decade or so about the intricate interrelationships among the body's many hormones and chemical processes.

Your thyroid might be functioning normally when examined independently, yet within the bigger picture of other hormone levels and functions, it becomes apparent that things aren't quite right. You might have a subtle adrenal gland imbalance (discussed in Chapter 8), or an immune system burdened with other challenges.

If your thyroid tests all come back with "normal" results, don't give up hope. Ask your doctor to explore other imbalances and health conditions that could affect, directly or indirectly, your thyroid's functions and your metabolism. Tests that are reasonable to request include those that help assess pituitary function, adrenal function, and immune function (such as anti-nuclear antibody, commonly elevated in autoimmune conditions such as rheumatoid arthritis). While continuing to explore possible causes for your symptoms, you might find it helpful to increase your dietary amounts of selenium (a trace mineral found in vegetables and animal-based foods, which your thyroid needs to convert T4 to T3), tyrosine (a protein found in meat and fish, which your thyroid needs to manufacture thyroid hormones), and iodine (a mineral found in seafood and iodized salt that your thyroid also needs to manufacture thyroid hormones). This might help you boost a slightly underactive thyroid's functions. It's important not to overdo it, of course, or you'll tip the balance in the other direction and could end up with overactive thyroid!

We discuss the relationships between the foods you eat and your thyroid's functions, and recommend healthy ways that you can influence thyroid balance through your diet and other lifestyle factors, in Chapter 15. If your doctor wants to settle on a diagnosis of chronic fatigue syndrome or fibromyalgia, based on your symptoms in addition to ruling out other clinical causes for them, ask your doctor to give you a trial of treatment with thyroid supplement. You have nothing to lose (but weight!) and everything (health and happiness!) to gain.

Part 2

Thyroid Conditions: Living out of Balance

6

Hypothyroidism:
Low and out of Balance

When your thyroid is underactive, you feel sluggish and under-active all over. You're tired and out of sorts, and numerous aches and discomforts seem to define your life. No matter what you eat or don't eat, you gain weight. You'd like to join the gym, but you don't even have enough energy to walk the dog. You can't get warm enough or remember things. Nothing is quite right, from your mood to your interest in activities that once gave you joy. Your body and your life are out of balance.

For the "lucky" two-thirds or so of you (quantifying the unknown is always a challenge), definitive lab results paint a clear clinical picture of hypothyroidism, and your doctor at least knows where to start with your treatment. Although the clinical thera-peutic path is straight and narrow, it will lead you to reason-able—and for some people, even complete—recovery. (Nearly everyone with thyroid imbalance benefits from an integrative approach that incorporates clinical and lifestyle methods, how-ever, which later chapters discuss.) As your metabolism returns to a state of balance, your symptoms gradually go away and you feel like yourself again. If you're among the lucky two-thirds, that is.

If you're among the one in three who isn't so lucky, your doctor doesn't know for sure what's going on with you. You've probably been through a battery of tests, none of which have revealed any abnormalities. You and your doctor both might suspect thyroid imbalance based on the symptoms that have brought you to seek treatment, but your lab results are either inconclusive or normal. All too often, doctors rule out thyroid problems on the basis of lab results alone. This is the legacy of conventional wisdom taught to them in medical school: body chemistry never lies. Well, true enough. *But it doesn't always tell the whole story, either.* Doctors have to connect the dots and fill in the spaces. And sometimes the picture a doctor paints from test results is the *wrong* picture.

DIAGNOSIS HYPOTHYROIDISM: SYMPTOMS AND CLINICAL FINDINGS

Nearly every doctor has seen patients who come in for symptoms of underactive thyroid and report histories of those symptoms going back as far as ten or twenty years. This is not because the patients were reluctant to seek medical care, but instead because they didn't realize that their problems and complaints were really health symptoms. Hindsight is always 20/20, as the cliché goes. Often, it's only in looking back that you can see the trail of discomforts and annoyances that now so clearly paint the picture of hypothyroidism. Underactive thyroid is so insidious, in fact, that there are as many (or more) people with *un*diagnosed or *mis*diagnosed hypothyroidism as there are with diagnosed hypothyroidism.

If your thyroid is underactive, you might feel that:

- It's especially hard to get out of bed in the morning, and to muster enough interest in the day's activities to participate in them.

- It's difficult to enjoy life because nothing seems worth the energy it takes to do it.
- You can't get warm enough, from your fingers and toes to the very core of your body.
- The muscles in your arms and legs ache and cramp, even when you're not using them.
- Your joints hurt.
- You can't concentrate, focus, or remember.
- You're somewhat "off," you're not yourself, but you can't explain, exactly, what that means.

These symptoms can be so strong that they interfere with your life, or so subtle that you don't realize you have them until someone (like your doctor) asks you specifically about them.

If your thyroid is underactive, your lab results might show:

- Low total T4 (less than 4.6)
- Low total T3 (less than 80)
- High TSH (over 5.5)
- High rT3, if tested
- Low radioactive iodine uptake (less than 10 percent), if tested
- Nothing out of the ordinary

When your lab results match your symptoms—that is, you fit both the clinical and chemical pictures—the diagnosis of hypothyroidism is easy enough. It's when you don't quite fit the pattern, which is more often than not the case, that it might take quite a while for your doctor to rule out any other problems before arriving at a diagnosis often presented to you as, "Well, I don't know what else it could be, so maybe it is your thyroid."

WHEN YOU HAVE ABNORMAL LAB RESULTS BUT NO SYMPTOMS

A surprising number of people don't have obvious symptoms of underactive thyroid, or have such mild symptoms that they don't recognize them as such, until blood tests during routine physical examination suggest hypothyroidism. There is always a bit of a dilemma when you have no symptoms but your lab tests point to an imbalance. Do you or do you not begin treatment? Many whose underactive thyroid is detected coincidently do benefit from treatment, physiologically in terms of how their bodies function as well as holistically in terms of how they feel. Only when treatment with thyroid supplement restores the balance of thyroid hormone in their bodies do they recognize that they hadn't been feeling up to par.

Most of the time, doctors want to treat underactive thyroid when lab tests show it is present, even if you're not experiencing any symptoms. This is because the potential for serious health problems, which we discuss a little later in this chapter, is so high when hypothyroidism is untreated. Also because of this potential, many health experts are now urging that blood tests for thyroid function be part of every routine physical examination. Can you safely choose to delay treatment if your blood tests show underactive thyroid but you have no symptoms? It depends.

Certainly you would want to repeat the blood tests, perhaps right away to verify the results (labs sometimes do make mistakes) and then every six months to monitor your thyroid hormone levels. Some of the integrative approaches that we'll discuss in later chapters might also influence your thyroid hormone levels enough to restore them to normal, if they are not significantly off. But odds are you're likely to feel better with treatment, even if you don't think you feel out of sorts now.

WHEN YOU HAVE SYMPTOMS BUT YOUR LAB RESULTS ARE NORMAL

A more frustrating problem for many people is having symptoms of underactive thyroid but normal lab results. We don't know why this happens, but we know that if you start thyroid treatment, your symptoms at least improve. The challenge for many people is convincing their doctors that they have underactive thyroid when the lab tests don't support such a diagnosis. Again, it's worth repeating the tests to verify the results. Normal values are ranges; individual sensitivities vary within those ranges. While one person with a TSH of 3 or a T4 of 8 might feel just fine, you might have the classic symptoms of underactive thyroid at the same values. Even though your test results are technically normal, your symptoms suggest that these values do not represent thyroid balance *for you*. If treatment with thyroid supplement drops your TSH to 1, barely above the low end of the range, and your symptoms lessen or go away, then your thyroid is underactive *for you*.

When you have symptoms of underactive thyroid but your thyroid tests all come back within normal ranges, it's important to also take a look at hypothalamic function, pituitary function, and adrenal function. Increasingly, doctors are finding that adrenal function in particular is the culprit when your symptoms paint one picture and your lab results paint another. Additional testing often can connect the two pictures for a more complete view of your endocrine function overall. Chapter 8 discusses adrenal function as it relates to thyroid function and the endocrine matrix.

FORMS AND CAUSES OF HYPOTHYROIDISM

There are numerous forms and causes of hypothyroidism. Doctors divide hypothyroidism into two camps: primary and secondary. In primary hypothyroidism, the thyroid gland malfunctions in some way, causing an imbalance of thyroid hormones and the resulting consequences throughout the metabolic matrix. In secondary hypothyroidism, the malfunction occurs beyond the thyroid, usually in what doctors call the HPT axis (hypothalamus-pituitary-thyroid interrelationship).

Treatment for secondary hypothyroidism targets the source of the malfunction, and may include thyroid supplementation as well. Treatment for primary hypothyroidism is generally the same—thyroid hormone supplement or replacement—regardless of form or cause. The chapters in Part 3 discuss conventional and alternative treatment approaches for primary hypothyroidism, as well as making treatment decisions.

GOITER

This rather odd word comes from the Latin word "guttur," which simply means "throat." A goiter actually is a symptom rather than a disease. It is a swelling of the thyroid gland that indicates your thyroid is straining to produce enough thyroid hormone. A goiter might also indicate that you're not getting enough iodine, although iodized salt has all but eliminated this cause in most Western countries (in the United States, iodized salt is mandated). Goiters are usually painless, although they can cause discomfort if they become large enough to press on other structures in your neck. When underactive thyroid is the cause of a goiter, the goiter usually goes away when treatment with thyroid supplement restores thyroid balance. When goiter is associated with iodine insufficiency, it's possible for blood thyroid hormone levels to be normal and for there to be no other symptoms of thyroid imbalance.

When goiter is associated with hypothyroidism:

- T3 and T4 are low
- TSH is elevated
- rT3 might be elevated, if tested
- Radioactive iodine uptake is low, if tested
- Goiter goes away when treatment restores
  thyroid balance

A goiter can manifest as a diffuse (overall) enlargement of the thyroid, or it can show up as a number of growths on the gland, in which case it's called a multinodular goiter.

A form of goiter called diffuse toxic goiter is associated with Graves' disease, a form of hyperthyroidism or overactive thyroid (see Chapter 7).

HASHIMOTO'S THYROIDITIS

Hashimoto's thyroiditis, named after the doctor who first identified it, is the most common cause of hypothyroidism. It is an autoimmune disease in which, for reasons we don't entirely understand, your body's immune system begins to perceive the tissue of your thyroid gland as foreign. Your immune system then sends cells to attack your thyroid gland, causing inflammation and swelling (goiter). The effect on your thyroid function might be first overactivity and then underactivity, although the end result is hypothyroidism as your immune system's attack on thyroid tissue disables the gland's ability to produce thyroid hormone. This damage and the resulting hypothyroidism are permanent. Chapter 9 explores the autoimmune connection to underactive and overactive thyroid.

When Hashimoto's thyroiditis is the cause of your hypothyroidism, typically your lab results will show:

- T3 and T4 are low
- TSH is elevated
- rT3 might be elevated (if your doctor requests this test)
- Radioactive iodine uptake is low (if your doctor requests this test)
- Antithyroid microsomal antibodies, antithyroglobulin antibodies, and anti-TPO antibodies are present (if your doctor requests any of these tests)

Your doctor might not test for the presence of antibodies because their presence or absence doesn't affect treatment. Because the hypothyroidism that results from Hashimoto's thyroiditis is permanent, treatment is lifelong thyroid supplementation. Hashimoto's thyroiditis is more common in people who already have other autoimmune disorders, particularly rheumatoid arthritis and type 1 diabetes (also called juvenile onset or insulin dependent diabetes).

HYPOTHYROIDISM FOLLOWING THYROIDECTOMY

The standard course of treatment for certain thyroid problems, such as cancer of the thyroid and severe Graves' disease, is surgery to remove all or a part of the gland. Once this is done, of course, the thyroid gland no longer functions (or it functions at a much reduced level that is inadequate for meeting your body's thyroid hormone needs). Sometimes radiation, such as to treat medical conditions involving structures of the throat or neck (cancer treatment), causes thyroid tissues to die and the thyroid gland to stop functioning. The end result is the same as if the thyroid gland had been surgically removed.

Whenever the thyroid gland stops functioning, you need to take thyroid hormone supplement. Thyroid hormones are essential for many body functions, including those that sustain life. Chapter 14 discusses the consequences of inadequate or no thyroid hormone in your body.

MYXEDEMIC COMA

Rarely, untreated hypothyroidism can cause a life-threatening crisis called myxedemic coma. Myxedema is an old term for hypothyroidism, and refers to the tissue swelling that is common with underactive thyroid. Without prompt diagnosis and treatment (immediate intravenous injection of thyroxine), myxedemic coma rather quickly leads to death. This complication comes on rapidly, progressing from complaints of feeling cold and drowsy to seizures and unconsciousness within hours. Body temperature can drop well below 85°F—a critical level.

Usually there is a precipitating event such as illness or injury that sends the body into crisis. Because the untreated hypothyroidism has altered cell metabolism, the body cannot muster the resources to respond to the crisis. It enters survival mode and begins to shut down functions. With rapid and appropriate emergency treatment followed by ongoing thyroid hormone replacement, you can recover from myxedemic coma without permanent consequences.

POSTPARTUM HYPOTHYROIDISM

It is fairly common for women to develop hypothyroidism during or immediately following pregnancy. This could have to do with the surge of hormones a woman's body experiences during pregnancy, or the strain pregnancy places on the thyroid gland to increase its activities to meet the changing needs of the woman's body. Most doctors recommend thyroid supplement treatment to make sure the woman's thyroid hormone blood levels stay within normal ranges.

Many women find that their thyroid functions return to normal when the hormones related to pregnancy and lactation return to normal, while others have permanent hypothyroidism. Some women do have continuing hypothyroidism. This is most likely to happen when there is a family history of thyroid imbalance or of autoimmune conditions. Thyroid hormones play a crucial role in brain development: if thyroid hormone levels are too low to meet the developing fetus's needs, permanent brain damage (intellectual impairment) results. In the United States this is a very rare problem because most doctors check the mother's thyroid levels at least once during each trimester (if the woman is receiving regular prenatal care). In parts of the world where natural iodine sources are limited, however, inadequate thyroid hormone levels during pregnancy is the leading cause of mental retardation.

In addition to ordering lab tests that measure TSH and T4/T3 levels, your doctor might order a thyroid microsomal autoantibodies (MSA) titer, which measures the ratio of these antibodies in your blood. Very low and very high MSA titers are good predictors of whether postpartum thyroid imbalance is likely to be a problem for you. A very low titer, less than 1:100, indicates very little antibody presence and little chance that hypothyroidism will develop. A very high titer, over 1:6400, indicates a high presence of antibodies and an increased likelihood that the underlying autoimmune process will produce hypothyroidism. Midrange titers seem to be neutral and aren't very helpful in predicting underactive thyroid.

There also appears to be a strong connection between a woman's estrogen and thyroid hormone levels. Hypothyroidism is more common in women at times when estrogen levels fluctuate, such as during pregnancy and menopause. The genes that researchers recently identified as holding thyroid receptors within the cell are also estrogen receptors. And some studies suggest direct correlations between T3 and T4 levels and estrogen levels. Researchers have observed that T3 and T4 levels drop in women who begin taking birth control pills or hormone replacement therapy (HRT).

UNDERACTIVE THYROID AND YOUR BRAIN

We are only now beginning to understand the connections between intellect, memory, emotions, and thyroid function. As many as half of those diagnosed with a form of mental illness, from depression and anxiety to bipolar disorder and schizo-phrenia, have low thyroid function. Doctors are now starting thyroid supplement treatment along with medications that treat the mental illness. For many people, a return to thyroid balance is also a return to emotional balance.

The symptoms of depression and the symptoms of under-active thyroid overlap: lethargy, disinterest in regular activities, fatigue. Depression and hypothyroidism might both be present, or one might be masking the other. If thyroid tests come back that support underactive thyroid, then your doctor will prob-ably start treatment with thyroid hormone supplement. Sometimes doctors will do a trial of thyroid treatment even if lab results are inconclusive or normal. If all of your symptoms then go away, hypothyroidism rather than depression is likely their cause. It is important to distinguish the underlying cause—hypothyroidism or depression—because both can have significant health ramifications.

HYPOTHYROIDISM AND AGING

While hypothyroidism can affect people of all ages, it becomes more common with increasing age. Studies suggest that as many as four in ten women over age 65 have underactive thyroid glands, often without symptoms other than abnormal lab test results. There are two dimensions to hypothyroidism and aging: how aging affects hypothyroidism, and how hypothyroidism affects aging.

How Aging Affects Hypothyroidism

When your body ages, it functions less efficiently. You might notice this as a sense that it takes you longer to get going, or that you move more slowly than you did when you were younger. Most all of us complain about these changes to some extent! Part of what happens is that the mitochondria begin to slow. They don't produce as much energy as they once did, and cell functions slow as a result.

One theory is that this allows free radicals (unattached molecules that attach themselves wherever they find molecules that can accept them) to increase, which in turn further decreases mitochondrial efficiency. Your body's needs for thyroid hormone increase to try to offset these changes. Eventually this demand exceeds your thyroid's ability to meet it, and you become hypothyroid.

How Hypothyroidism Affects Aging

One function encoded in mitochondrial DNA is apoptosis, or programmed cell death. This is the point and rate at which cells die off. While we know this rate increases with age, we don't know precisely how mitochondrial function regulates it. Some researchers speculate that hypothyroidism, because of its effect on mitochondrial respiration, speeds up apoptosis to increase the rate of cell death. Cells that function less efficiently are a liability for the body, so it attempts to get rid of them. So not only does hypothyroidism increase with age, but also it might contribute to an accelerated aging process.

More certain are the effects underactive thyroid has on body functions such as fatty acid metabolism and mental health. Low thyroid hormone levels interfere with your body's ability to break down LDL ("bad" cholesterol). As LDL levels rise, so does your risk for heart disease. If you have high blood-cholesterol levels and also have some of the symptoms of underactive thyroid, it's worth having your doctor do some thyroid tests.

There's increasing evidence that some of the memory loss and dementia we associate with aging is neither inevitable nor untreatable. Thyroid hormone levels affect brain function in many ways, from its role in nerve cell metabolism to its interactions with neurotransmitters and other hormones. Many older people with memory and cognitive problems also have underactive thyroid. Restoring thyroid balance restores brain functions, improving both memory and cognition. Of course, there are many causes for disturbances to these functions that have nothing to do with thyroid function, including diseases such as Alzheimer's and Parkinson's.

CAN YOU PREVENT HYPOTHYROIDISM?

Hypothyroidism is the most common thyroid disorder in most parts of the world. To some degree, preventing it is simply a matter of making sure you get enough iodine in your diet. Your thyroid gland uses iodine to manufacture thyroid hormones. You don't need much iodine, which is a natural element found in the soil. In many parts of the world, however, the iodine content of soil is poor, so food plants grown in it do not contain enough dietary iodine to meet the body's needs. Iodized salt has prevented millions of cases of hypothyroidism that would otherwise result.

The Human Genome Project offers much promise that in the future we will find ways to delay or prevent hypothyroidism not related to iodine intake. Some of this research focuses on genetic factors, and other research targets lifestyle factors such as nutrition and exercise. We talk more about these factors in later chapters.

7

Hyperthyroidism: High and out of Balance

When your thyroid gland is overactive, you feel like someone's kicked your body and your life into overdrive. You have more energy than you can possibly use, which makes it hard for you to fall asleep at night. You feel jittery, hyped up, like there's a continual infusion of caffeine flowing into your veins. Your heart pounds and occasionally seems to miss a few beats, acting as though it keeps getting ahead of itself. And while at first it wasn't so bad to drop a few pounds without trying, now your friends are asking if you're okay in those hushed tones people use when they fear the answer will be "no." You aren't okay, of course; it's not normal for your heart to feel like it's coming right out of your chest and for your brain to be so busy you can't get any rest. You're concerned, maybe even frightened, so you schedule an appointment with your doctor for as soon as you can get in.

The differences between hyperthyroidism and hypothyroidism are marked and dramatic right from the start. While you might be able to go on for years feeling tired and unenergetic, as is the hallmark of hypothyroidism, you can't tolerate the sense that your body is ready to run away without you, as is the hallmark of hyperthyroidism. In most cases, when your thyroid is overactive, diagnosis and treatment are straightforward. Although your body can tolerate hypothyroidism for a surprisingly long time without permanent damage, it can deal with the stress of hyperthyroidism for only a short time before there is significant risk for damage to your heart, kidneys, bones, and eyes.

WHAT CAUSES HYPERTHYROIDISM

Although we don't know precisely *how* hyperthyroidism gets its start, there is not nearly as much mystery surrounding its causes as cloaks the causes and progression of hypothyroidism. In hyperthyroidism, the thyroid gland produces too much thyroid hormone. This happens as the result of:

- Graves' disease (also called toxic diffuse goiter)
- Toxic nodular goiter
- Thyroiditis (inflammation of the thyroid gland)
- Thyrotoxicosis factitiae (taking too much thyroid supplement)

Like hypothyroidism, hyperthyroidism is either primary (originating in the thyroid gland) or secondary (caused by dysfunctions elsewhere in the body, usually the pituitary or hypothalamus). Treating the underlying cause eliminates secondary hyperthyroidism. It doesn't appear that mitochondrial function has a particularly close connection to hyperthyroidism, except in situations in which there is a constellation of mitochondrial disorders. In such situations, there appears to be defects in the mitochondrial DNA that are responsible for the entire constellation of disorders, and the hyperthyroidism is likely to be secondary.

If your thyroid is overactive, you might feel that:

- No matter how tired you are, you can't fall asleep or stay asleep.

- You are always hot, sweaty, and flushed, no matter how cold the external temperature, and your body temperature might be slightly elevated (99°F).
- You are so hungry that you eat all the time, yet you're losing weight.
- You worry about everything (anxiety), and have wide mood swings.
- You are weak and your hands shake (tremors).
- Your heart races and seems to skip beats (palpitations).
- Your eyes are red, irritated, and look to others as though they are fixed in a blank stare.

Women with overactive thyroid often have irregular menstrual periods—you might have excessive bleeding one month, and then go several months without a period. The length of time it takes to develop symptoms with hyperthyroidism is fairly short compared to the often lengthy and insidious onset of hypothyroidism that typically takes place over months or even years. When your thyroid is overactive, your lab tests might show:

- Elevated total T4 (over 12)
- Elevated total T3 (over 180)
- Low or immeasurable TSH (under 0.5)
- Elevated serum thyroglobulin, if tested
- Low rT3, if tested
- High radioactive iodine uptake (more than 30 percent), if tested

If you have all the results supporting hyperthyroidism but your TSH is normal or elevated, this indicates that your hyperthyroidism is secondary to a TSH-secreting anterior pituitary tumor or to pituitary resistance to thyroid hormone (more about these situations in Chapter 8). If your lab results are normal, something other than hyperthyroidism is causing your symptoms. Lab results provide conclusive diagnosis of hyperthyroidism, unlike hypothyroidism.

GRAVES' DISEASE

Graves' disease, also called diffuse toxic goiter, is the most common form of hyperthyroidism, accounting for about 90 percent of all cases. It usually occurs in people between the ages of 20 and 40, although it is becoming increasingly common over age 65, and affects women eight times as often as men. About 2 percent of women in the United States become diagnosed with Graves' disease. The most prominent feature associated with Graves' disease is goiter, an overall swelling of the thyroid gland that occurs as the thyroid takes in far more iodine than it can convert to thyroid hormone. The goiter is considered "toxic" because it is producing a harmful level of thyroid hormones, and diffuse because it infiltrates the entire thyroid gland.

Graves' disease is an autoimmune disorder in which your body's immune system produces antibodies that attack the tissues of your thyroid gland—specifically, the TSH receptors. Once destroyed by antibodies, these receptors can no longer function to keep T4 and T3 production in check, so your thyroid gland just keeps pouring these hormones out into your bloodstream. It's like having a stuck accelerator in your car, continually flooding the engine with gasoline. The T4 converts to T3 at a rapid rate to maintain the proper balance between the two forms of thyroid hormone. The abundant T3 binds with available cell receptors (and T2 with mitochondrial receptors), effectively turbocharging your metabolism. Some doctors also call Graves' disease thyrotoxicosis, which is a bit confusing but simply means "poisoning of the thyroid." This is not the same problem as thyrotoxicosis factitiae, which we'll discuss later in this chapter.

Graves' disease is chronic, which means it will come and go over the course of a long period of time (probably the rest of your life). The severity of symptoms fluctuates. Although doctors generally start out treating Graves' disease with drugs called antithyroids that suppress thyroid hormone production, for most people this is only a temporary solution. Eventually the thyroid gland becomes resistant to the effects of these drugs, and thyroid hormone production creeps back up. Doctors usually recommend a course of radioactive iodine to permanently damage the thyroid gland to stop it from producing thyroid hormone altogether, or if that fails, surgery to remove part or all of the thyroid gland. While both of these treatments "fix" the problem of hyperthyroidism, they create the new problem of *hypo*thyroidism, which will then require ongoing treatment and management. (More about the treatment methods for hyperthyroidism later in this chapter.)

There are two conditions that can develop as a result of Graves' disease, and that after developing run a course independent from the Graves' disease. Both are autoimmune situations in which antibodies different from those that cause Graves' disease attack either the structures of the eyes or of the skin.

The first is infiltrative ophthalmopathy, the symptoms of which include pain and irritation in and around the eye, excessive tearing, sensitivity to light (photophobia), "bulging" eyes (exophthalmos), and damage to the muscles that support the eye. This damage weakens the eye muscles to the extent that they can no longer control the eye's movements, resulting in double vision. Infiltrative ophthalmopathy requires treatment separate from that for Graves' disease.

In cases of infiltrative dermopathy (also called pretibial myxedema), lesions form on the shins. These lesions are itchy and inflamed at first, and then heal into leathery patches. They can appear long after Graves' disease is under control.

There is as yet no way to prevent Graves' disease, or even to predict who might be at increased risk for developing it. Graves' disease does seem to run in families, which suggests a genetic link of some sort, but researchers haven't been able to identify it. Early identification and treatment remain the most effective way to prevent Graves' disease from having serious consequences.

TOXIC NODULAR GOITER

In toxic nodular goiter, only part of the thyroid gland is enlarged. This can be because of a single nodule or multiple nodules that are isolated. When examining your neck, your doctor will feel one or more lumps rather than an overall swelling of your thyroid gland. The vast majority of thyroid nodules—more than 95 percent—are benign, or noncancerous. The most efficient and effective test of thyroid nodules is fine needle aspiration biopsy, in which the doctor inserts a thin needle into the nodule, withdraws a sample of cells, and examines them under the microscope. Toxic nodular goiters become more common as you get older.

Treatment options for noncancerous nodules include:

- Iodine (not radioactive)
- Radioactive iodine
- Surgery to remove the nodule

Antithyroid drugs usually aren't effective in treating toxic nodular goiter. Treatment for cancerous nodules is specific to the nature of the nodule and might include surgery, radiation therapy, radioactive iodine, or other approaches.

THYROIDITIS

Thyroiditis is an inflammation of the thyroid gland. The inflammation can be viral, autoimmune (as in Graves' disease), bacterial, or idiopathic (of unknown origin). Thyroiditis, except for Graves' disease, often goes away on its own or with just short-term antithyroid drug treatment. Hashimoto's thyroiditis, the most common form of *hypo*thyroidism, is an inflammation that starts with hyperthyroidism. However, the hyperthyroid phase is so short that you might not even notice it before the symptoms of hypothyroidism set in. Watchful waiting is often a prudent course of action to take. Sometimes, swallowing is affected. If the inflammation is causing discomfort or unusual swelling, sometimes corticosteroid anti-inflammatory drugs or nonsteroidal anti-inflammatory drugs (NSAIDs) can provide relief. Most nonautoimmune cases of thyroiditis eventually go away without any residual symptoms or need for ongoing treatment. Autoimmune thyroiditis, such as Graves' disease or Hashimoto's thyroiditis, nearly always requires continuing medical treatment.

THYROTOXICOSIS FACTITIAE

Thyrotoxicosis factitiae ("not natural") results from taking too much thyroid hormone supplement, usually when treating hypothyroidism. Treatment may or may not be necessary, depending on the kind of symptoms you have. A large overdose could result in a thyroid storm, a potentially life-threatening hyperthyroid crisis (more on this in a later section of this chapter). Most of the time, treatment consists of adjusting the thyroid hormone supplement dose and monitoring blood thyroid hormone levels until they are stable. If you are taking thyroid hormone supplements, especially forms containing short-acting T3, have your blood levels checked once a year and whenever you notice symptoms that could be overactive thyroid.

HYPERTHYROIDISM AND THE METABOLIC MATRIX

The effects of hyperthyroidism on other body systems can be sudden, dramatic, and dangerous. Thyroid hormone stimulates the release of ACTH, the "stress" hormone. ACTH causes a multitude of "fight-or-flight" reactions to take place, including increased heart rate and breathing, raised blood pressure, and increased body temperature. Your body can sustain this heightened state for only so long before it begins to experience tissue and cell damage. Two serious heart conditions, atrial fibrillation and tachycardia, can develop. These might require treatment to prevent further damage and heart failure, until your hyperthyroidism is under control.

Overactive thyroid affects the metabolic matrix in other ways. Increased cell metabolism signals the pancreas to produce more insulin, so cells can "burn" more energy in the form of glucose (blood sugar). It also affects the metabolism of fatty acids, decreasing conversion of sugars to fats for stored energy supplies. And it alters vitamin metabolism.

BONE DENSITY AND OSTEOPOROSIS

Overactive thyroid draws calcium from your bones into your bloodstream, partly as a function of altered vitamin metabolism and partly to meet the increased needs your body has for calcium since your cardiac system is running in high gear. Calcium is one of the electrolytes your heart muscle uses to carry electrical impulses through heart tissues, causing your heart to contract. Your body stores extra calcium in your bones, and then "withdraws" it when demand exceeds supply. The result can quickly escalate to osteoporosis, a dangerous thinning and weakening of the bone. This leaves you vulnerable to spontaneous fractures, particularly in the spine, wrists, hips, and ankles. It doesn't take long for hyperthyroidism to take your bone density to an unsafe level. Many doctors will do a bone density scan, which is quick and painless, on all women whom they diagnosis with hyperthyroidism, and on men who are 65 or older. Bone density naturally decreases with age. Because women have less bone mass than men do to start with, their rate of loss is more significant.

THYROID STORM

Thyroid storm, also called thyrotoxic crisis or thyrotoxic storm, is a hyperthyroidism attack that comes on strongly and suddenly. It is a life-threatening emergency; without immediate treatment, it can result in death in a matter of hours. Symptoms include fever (which can shoot as high as 106°F), extreme restlessness and mood swings, enlarged liver, jaundice, confusion, psychosis, and coma. Generally hyperthyroidism has been present but untreated or undertreated, and there is some sort of event, such as illness, injury, or surgery, that limits the body's ability to accommodate the additional stress and sets off the thyroid storm. Treatment includes immediate intravenous antithyroid drugs and drugs to stabilize blood pressure and heart rate.

APATHETIC HYPERTHYROIDISM

The elderly, particularly those who have already experienced significant loss of function, may develop a form of hyperthyroidism that is insidious and frequently undetected. This form, sometimes called apathetic hyperthyroidism, actually looks more like underactive thyroid at first glance. The person becomes tired; less engaged in the world, as if depressed (which is how this form of overactive thyroid gets the name "apathetic"); and can become confused or agitated. The typical findings of hyperthyroidism, such as heat intolerance and rapid heart rate, are often missing. Blood tests for thyroid hormone levels, however, may reveal the existence of hyperactive thyroid. Treatment of this form of hyperthyroidism is the same as for any other form of overactive thyroid, although it's important to proceed with great caution, as the older a person is, the more sensitive the body is to drugs.

TREATMENTS FOR HYPERTHYROIDISM

There are three general treatment paths for hyperthyroidism:

- Antithyroid drugs
- Radioactive iodine
- Surgery

Antithyroid drugs provide temporary relief of overactive thyroid symptoms, while radioactive iodine and surgery permanently destroy and remove, respectively, the thyroid gland. Chapter 11 discusses treatments for overactive thyroid more extensively.

ANTITHYROID DRUGS

The two antithyroid drugs doctors most commonly prescribe are propylthiouracil (PTU) and methimazole (also known as the brand-name drug Tapazole). These drugs work by preventing your thyroid gland from producing and releasing thyroid hormone. PTU also interferes with the conversion of T4 to T3. The usual therapeutic approach is to take one drug or the other for up to two years, by which time your hyperthyroidism (usually Graves' disease) has gone into remission. Repeat courses of therapy are sometimes necessary.

Both of these drugs have potentially serious side effects involving the liver, and are not usually prescribed if you have liver disease or liver function problems of any kind, or if you are pregnant or could become pregnant. About four in ten people with hyperthyroidism who receive antithyroid drug treatment will return to normal thyroid function. The remainder will find that their symptoms return within a year or two of ending treatment, and will need multiple courses of antithyroid drug therapy or a different treatment approach.

RADIOACTIVE IODINE

Radioactive sodium iodine, I^{131}, is the most common and most effective treatment for hyperthyroidism, particularly Graves' disease. It works by killing cells in the thyroid gland, ending their ability to produce thyroid hormone. Unfortunately, dosing is less than precise and about half of those who receive this treatment end up with underactive thyroid because the I^{131} completely shuts down thyroid hormone production in the thyroid gland. Although many people who undergo radioactive iodine treatment worry that it will cause cancer, there so far are no studies that support this. Radioactive iodine seems a safe and effective treatment for hyperthyroidism, with the most serious side effect being hypothyroidism following treatment.

SURGERY

Surgery removes part or all of the thyroid gland, depending on the reason for your hyperthyroidism. In most cases, it is the treatment of last resort, used only when antithyroid drugs and radioactive iodine either have failed or are not practical. The surgeon makes an incision following one of the skin folds or lines in the neck to help mask the scar after it heals, and tries to remove no more of the thyroid gland than is necessary.

One difficulty with thyroid surgery actually has more to do with the parathyroid glands, the small glands that lie above the thyroid and (along with calcitonin, a thyroid hormone) control calcium metabolism. Extensive thyroid surgery may affect these glands, resulting in calcium abnormalities.

OVERACTIVE THYROID AND YOUR BRAIN

Too much thyroid hormone in your body makes you feel "revved up" all the time. This often involves heightened brain activity. You might feel anxious, and even have delusions or feelings of paranoia. Generally, if these symptoms are related to thyroid imbalance rather than other causes, they will go away with treatment for hyperthyroidism. Overactive thyroid is not as likely as underactive thyroid to be the cause of mental health problems.

WHAT CAN YOU DO TO PREVENT HYPERTHYROIDISM?

The only form of hyperthyroidism that you can prevent is that caused by taking too much thyroid hormone supplement to treat hypothyroidism. If you have underactive thyroid and are taking thyroid hormone supplement, you should have T3, T4, and TSH levels drawn once a year after your dose stabilizes, and whenever you experience a significant change in your health condition (including weight loss or gain). Eating larger-than-normal amounts of certain foods can increase your thyroid gland's thyroid hormone production, including:

- Soy products (in moderate amounts; high amounts can have the opposite effect of suppressing thyroid function)
- Vegetables grown in iodine-rich soil

Whether or not you're taking treatment for hypothyroidism, if you notice any of the symptoms of overactive thyroid, see your doctor without delay.

8

Sluggish Thyroid, Stressful Adrenal?

Doctors are beginning to believe that it is nearly impossible for thyroid imbalance, particularly underactive thyroid, to exist without a corresponding imbalance in adrenal function. This reflects new understanding and a shift in perspective regarding the interrelationships among the structures of the endocrine matrix.

For about one in two of you reading this book because you have a thyroid imbalance—50 percent—the source of your body's imbalance extends beyond the functions of your thyroid gland to involve the interplay among your thyroid gland and other endocrine structures. Five endocrine structures that work closely together are the hypothalamus, pituitary gland, adrenal glands, thyroid gland, and sex glands (ovaries or testes). Conventional medicine views the interactions of these structures as two parallel cycles, commonly identified as the HPA axis and the HPT axis. The HPA axis contains the hypothalamus, pituitary, and adrenals. The HPT axis contains the hypothalamus, pituitary, and thyroid. The conventional view portrays each axis as a fairly independent cycle of feedback loops and action/reaction chains, with occasional points of cross-contact.

As our understanding of the intricacies and complexities of endocrine functions within the body increases, however, it is becoming clear that these axes are not linear alignments that only interact intermittently and under certain circumstances. Rather, their elements are constantly communicating and continually adjusting to each other as well as to other activities and functions throughout your body. And rather than linear links or cause-and-effect actions, this is a web of connections, some intimate and some distant but all nonetheless "touching" in some way. It is because of these interrelationships that imbalance in one area nearly always results in, or reflects, imbalance in other areas. Each structure within the endocrine matrix has specialized and unique functions, but does not carry them out in isolation or without affecting the functions of the others.

It's a constantly changing matrix. Think of yourself treading water at the beach. All four limbs are in constant motion, speeding up or slowing down each stroke according to what they sense is necessary to keep you afloat. Meanwhile, each breath adjusts to your need for oxygen, and to the waves that splash over you. Your eyes receive information about waves about to hit you, and your body's movements respond instantaneously. And all the while, you are receiving the sensations of a lovely beach day, enjoying these sensations, and perhaps holding a conversation with those in the water around you. In the same way, your endocrine matrix functions in a rhythm of constantly coordinated motion and activity.

NEW THINKING: STRESS AND YOUR METABOLIC MATRIX

Stress defines your life. Not that you need a book to tell you this, of course. Deadlines, traffic, kids, what to make for dinner—you know stress. But what your body views as stress and what you're thinking of right now as stress are sometimes different. In its simplest definition, stress is any event or situation that requires a change. Stress can be physical or emotional, positive or negative—and often is a combination. Whatever its nature, stress affects just about every function of your body to some degree. Although we tend to think of stress as a bad thing, a certain amount of it is necessary.

WHAT IS STRESS?

From your body's perspective, stress is what keeps things running. Just as tension makes it possible for a violin string to make music, stress makes the functions of living possible. Press the string, change the tone, let the music come forth. When stress becomes constant rather than episodic, however, it becomes dysfunctional—that is, it causes normal body functions to become abnormal. Place too much stress on the violin string, and it snaps. Put too much stress on your body's systems, and they struggle. It's easy enough to replace the violin string. But damage to body systems can be far-reaching—and permanent, if you don't intervene to bring it under control.

Physical stress ranges from the sequence of events that take place every time you put one foot in front of the other to walk to the subtle adaptations your cells make in reaction to the thousands of chemical and electrical signals they receive every minute. Physical stress can come in the form of exercise and activity, surgery and drugs, or injury, illness, and infection. Even the foods you eat can be sources of physical stress for your body, for the nutrition that they do or do not supply. Imbalances in your body, such as those that result from underactive or overactive thyroid, are also forms of physical stress. Emotional stress arises from the experiences you have each day, and affects the physical functions of your body. Emotional stress can cause you to feel happy, sad, angry, frustrated, fatigued, or "stressed out." Some of these effects (or their consequences) are easy to observe, such as laughing or crying. Others take place well within your body, and do not become apparent until they cause significant physical changes.

THE PHYSIOLOGY OF STRESS:
THE FIGHT-OR-FLIGHT MATRIX

Faster than you can snap your fingers, your body responds to a stress event with a network of actions and reactions. Your hypothalamus shoots corticotropin-releasing hormone (CRH) to your pituitary gland, which in turn sends adrenocorticotropic hormone (ACTH) racing to your adrenal glands. This is like sending mild-mannered Clark Kent, Superman's alter ego, into the phone booth. A few blurred spins and suddenly there's the man of steel himself, stronger than a locomotive and faster than a speeding bullet. Ordinarily your adrenal glands have a low-key, Clark Kent kind of existence. They're content to busy themselves generating the hormones that regulate such humdrum functions as converting fat and other nutrients into forms your body can use and making sure your levels of testosterone (in men) or progesterone (in women) are adequate. But then there's a crisis, and out from your adrenals surge the superpower hormones:

- Epinephrine (also called adrenaline), which causes your heart to beat harder and faster, dilates (opens) your airways so each breath brings in more oxygen, and constricts (narrows) the blood vessels serving nonvital organs to make more blood available to vital organs.
- Norepinephrine, which causes major blood vessels to constrict to increase blood pressure.
- Cortisol, which increases insulin sensitivity. This allows cells to "burn" more sugar, increasing their energy output and making possible an intensified but short-term physical response such as running.

It seems a bit extreme to set all of this in motion just because you hit your thumb with a hammer, or a careless driver nearly crashes into you at an intersection. But this stress response role in the CRH-ACTH-cortisol matrix is really the primary purpose of your adrenal glands. From studying the remains of primitive humans excavated from archeological sites around the world, researchers know that the structure of the adrenal glands has changed little in the 10,000 years or so of human existence. And in the beginning, the fight-or-flight response that commandeered the body in times of stress often was the difference between life and death. When a cornered mastodon turned on those hunting it, the hunters became the hunted. Survival was a matter of fight or flight, pure and simple.

Life in our modern times is neither pure nor simple, of course. And it's been thousands of years since we worried more about becoming dinner than fixing dinner. But our bodies still carry that primal fight-or-flight response in reaction to stress. And even though we're no longer slaying mastodons, the stresses of modern everyday life continue to activate the stress response.

STRESS AND ADRENAL FUNCTION

Stress affects adrenal function in two ways. First, there is a constantly elevated stress response and cortisol secretion. The adrenal gland is forever pumping its hormones into the bloodstream. As a consequence, the signs and symptoms of high cortisol develop: high blood sugar, poor sleep, increased fat stores, decreased healing, and osteopenia (weakened bones). And second, the feedback mechanism designed to let the hypothalamus and pituitary know to stop stimulating the adrenal gland becomes malfunctional and ineffective.

With so many stimuli bombarding this mechanism originally designed to preserve survival, it doesn't take long for your adrenal glands to become overwhelmed. The baseline of the rise-and-fall cycle of neurotransmitters and hormones rises, and the cycle itself flattens out. The adrenals function in crisis mode for so long that it becomes the "normal" state. Because they cannot continue to function in such a way, they then stop responding to stress. As a result, you feel fatigued and unenergetic. Your body no longer has the adrenal resources to kick your metabolism into a higher gear, no matter what stresses you face. This taxes other structures in your endocrine matrix as they try to make up the difference, and also taxes other body systems.

ADRENAL FATIGUE

Clinically speaking, adrenal fatigue is the state that results when the lab tests that measure adrenal function come back within normal limits but you have symptoms of underactive adrenal function. It's not quite a disease state, but it's not a state of normal function, either. Your adrenal glands still produce the hormones and neurotransmitters they are supposed to produce, but they don't give you the boost that you need when stress strikes, either. They've "tapped out" at a higher baseline, so it takes more to kick up the levels.

THE ADRENAL-THYROID CONNECTION

Conservative estimates are that half of people diagnosed with hypothyroidism also have adrenal fatigue. Answering these questions can help you decide if you might be among them:

Do you wake up feeling refreshed and invigorated after a sufficiently long night's sleep (six to eight hours), or are you still groggy and irritable?

Do you feel more tired or less tired as your day goes on?

Are you irritable, moody, and anxious regardless of events taking place around you?

Do you have heart palpitations (irregular and rapid beats)?

Is your blood pressure high or low?

Do you startle easily?

Do you crave salt or salty foods?

Do you seem to get sick with every virus that makes the rounds?

Do you easily gain weight or have trouble losing weight?

Do your eyes look puffy and swollen, like you've been crying, or dark and sunken, like you haven't slept for days?

Do you feel lightheaded when you get up after lying down or sitting?

Are you currently taking thyroid hormone supplement (T4) for underactive thyroid?

There are no right or wrong answers to these questions, and your answers aren't necessarily conclusive. But they might give you insight into how far-reaching your body's imbalance is. Here's what your answers suggest:

People with adrenal fatigue tend to wake up groggy and irritable, feeling that they didn't get enough sleep no matter how many hours of sleep they did get.

When your primary imbalance is thyroid, you're likely to feel more tired as the day goes on. When adrenal fatigue is a factor, you might feel better the longer you're awake and up.

Irritability and mood swings are common with both adrenal fatigue and thyroid imbalance. Anxiety is more likely to accompany adrenal fatigue or overactive thyroid.

Heart palpitations, or feelings that your heart is going to burst out of your chest, are common with overactive thyroid and adrenal fatigue.

Low blood pressure is common with adrenal fatigue. This is a combination result from decreased cortisol and reduced fluid volume.

When your adrenal glands are taxed to the point at which they're no longer responding appropriately to stresses that you encounter, you feel like your nerves are on edge. This is the result of erratic cortisol levels and disturbances in your cortisol production cycle. In this heightened state, your body is programmed to respond literally in a heartbeat.

Another of the hormones your adrenal glands produce is aldosterone, one action of which is to regulate the amount of salt that your kidneys filter from your blood. When your hypothalamus perceives stress, it secretes CRH to initiate the CRH-ACTH-cortisol matrix. If your adrenals are in a state of fatigue and are no longer responding appropriately to the call for cortisol, your pituitary perceives this as an unanswered need and continues sending ACTH anyway. This in turn stimulates your adrenals to pump up production of aldosterone, which draws even more salt from your body. Your body sends you signals to increase salt ingestion—so you crave salt.

Cortisol is essential for helping your body to heal. When your cortisol response becomes inadequate, your immune system lacks the full range of resources it needs to keep you healthy. This lowers your resistance, leaving you vulnerable to infections and inflammations.

Weight gain is common when the problem is underactive thyroid. You also can get weight gain from chronically high cortisol levels due to the elevated insulin and blood sugar.

When your adrenal glands are fatigued, this affects their production of aldosterone, which directs how your kidneys excrete salt. This pulls fluid back from the skin and tissues just beneath it, causing your face and especially the area around your eyes to look sunken. With underactive thyroid, fluid tends to collect in the face and around the eyes as a result of slowed metabolism.

A condition called orthostatic hypotension—positional low blood pressure—is a common and early symptom of adrenal fatigue.

If you're taking thyroid supplement for underactive thyroid and you still have the symptoms of hypothyroidism, there's a good chance that other components of your endocrine matrix are out of balance, too.

The symptoms of adrenal fatigue are often difficult to distinguish from those of thyroid imbalance, especially underactive thyroid. They include:

- Exhaustion and fatigue upon waking that seems to improve as the day goes on
- Feeling faint when sitting up after lying down or standing after sitting
- Difficulty falling asleep or staying asleep
- Muscle and joint pain
- Lack of energy
- Lethargy and apathy
- Feeling cold regardless of environmental temperature

Adrenal fatigue does not cause thyroid imbalance, but it does intensify the symptoms of underactive thyroid. When these symptoms persist even after you begin thyroid hormone supplements to treat underactive thyroid, it's worth having your doctor follow up with adrenal function tests as well as repeat thyroid hormone tests.

TESTING ADRENAL FUNCTION

There are various ways to test adrenal function: blood tests, adrenal stress tests, urine tests, and saliva tests designed to stimulate adrenal function. Blood tests usually look at blood electrolyte levels, or the amounts and balances of salts in your blood, and the levels of the hormones renin and ACTH. Conventional medicine looks at a morning cortisol level, but this measurement usually is normal unless there is frank adrenal insufficiency, called Addison's disease. This will not usually pick up the subtler findings of adrenal exhaustion. A more specific test is the ACTH stimulation test, in which an injection of ACTH is given, and blood tested for cortisol at baseline and at subsequent intervals, usually one-half hour and one hour. Although there are many interpretations of this test, we generally will suspect adrenal exhaustion if the cortisol does not double within one hour. This tells us that the adrenal does not respond as swiftly to a pituitary hormone stimulus. Another way of doing this test is by giving you an injection of ACTH and then measuring how much cortisol you excrete in urine collected over 24 hours.

Adrenal hormones have a natural ebb and flow throughout the day, being highest in the morning and lowest at night. Saliva tests involve collecting saliva samples at certain intervals over 24 hours, which provides "snapshots" that present the fluctuations of adrenal hormones. Because a blood test is an "artificial" situation, many doctors rely on saliva tests to give a fuller picture of the adrenal function throughout a 24-hour period.

TREATING ADRENAL FATIGUE

Doctors are now starting to treat adrenal fatigue and its cascading consequences with low doses of hydrocortisone given over a short period of time, from seven days up to three or four months. This seems to restore balance along the CRH-ACTH-cortisol matrix, giving the adrenal glands a much-needed break from the pattern of continual response that has trapped them for so long. Adding hydrocortisone, a drug that is identical to the body's own hormone, to the body's own supply raises the circulating levels of cortisol enough to turn off the pituitary's ACTH signals and the CRH signals from the hypothalamus.

Many people with adrenal fatigue are already taking thyroid hormone supplement to treat underactive thyroid, which typically continues in conjunction with treatment with hydrocortisone. Adding low doses of T3 seems to further improve symptoms. Glycyrrhiza, an extract from licorice that you can buy at health-food stores, also can help. It slows the liver's metabolism of cortisol to keep more of it circulating in your bloodstream. Licorice belongs to a group of herbs called "adaptogens," so named for their ability to help the adrenal gland adapt to greater stress conditions without requiring more hormone secretion. Other adaptogenic herbs include Eleutherococcus (Siberian ginseng), Rhodiola rosea, and a fungus called Cordyceps. And of course, doing as much as possible to reduce the sources of stress in your life goes a long way toward easing the strain on your adrenal glands, your endocrine matrix, and your body in general.

Once adrenal fatigue seems to be under control, it's sometimes necessary to adjust the thyroid hormone supplement. Dietary and other lifestyle changes often are helpful (see Chapters 15, 16, and 19 for more information). Other autoimmune conditions that you might have, such as rheumatoid arthritis, might also improve as adrenal fatigue subsides.

BEYOND FATIGUE: ADDISON'S DISEASE

One of the most important purposes of testing adrenal function is to look for Addison's disease. This potentially serious condition occurs when there is damage of some kind to your adrenal glands that interferes with their ability to function. Most of the time Addison's disease is an autoimmune condition, although tumors and other diseases, most notably tuberculosis, can cause it as well. Addison's disease requires lifetime cortisol replacement and regular blood tests to monitor its stability.

Although Addison's disease is an uncommon disorder, already having one autoimmune condition involving an endocrine structure, such as hypothyroidism (or diabetes or rheumatoid arthritis) or type 2 diabetes, makes it more likely that you'll have another. Like tests for thyroid function, adrenal function tests are not always conclusive.

THE STRESS RESPONSE
AND YOUR SEX GLANDS

Most people don't consider the sex organs as part of the stress response, but they are a critical component of your metabolic matrix. The sex hormones and the adrenal hormones all come from the same source—cholesterol. When your body constantly calls for the formation of adrenaline and cortisol, there is less cholesterol available to form proper testosterone, estrogen, and progesterone. This is partly why chronic stress is associated with lack of sexual response, with abnormalities of menstruation, and with exhaustion. Even fertility is known to be affected by stress.

As well, the adrenal gland produces low amounts of the sex hormones. This isn't as critical when you're young, but at menopause the ovaries cease to produce these hormones. If the adrenal is fatigued, it has less energy to cushion this hormone depletion, resulting in severe menopausal symptoms caused by lack of estrogen and progesterone.

POLYGLANDULAR DEFICIENCY SYNDROME

It's not uncommon for more than one component of your endocrine matrix to fail to function properly. You might have hypothyroidism along with type 2 diabetes, adrenal fatigue, and pernicious anemia, for example. This situation is called polyglandular ("many glands") deficiency syndrome. Often, an autoimmune process damages the involved structures. Conditions that might appear in polyglandular deficiency syndrome include any combination of the following:

- Hashimoto's thyroiditis and other forms of hypothyroidism
- Graves' disease (a form of hyperthyroidism)
- Insulin-dependent diabetes (either type 1 or type 2 that requires insulin)
- Addison's disease
- Pernicious anemia
- Vitiligo
- Alopecia

These conditions can appear in any order and in any combination. In research settings, further immune system testing reveals compromised immune function at the T-cell level (more on this in Chapter 9) in about a third of people who have polyglandular deficiency syndrome. There also appears to be a genetic connection; immediate family members often have similar T-cell compromise as well as one or more endocrine disorders. Treatment focuses on supplying your body with enough of the deficient hormones to restore balance to your endocrine matrix.

WILSON'S RT3 DOMINANCE SYNDROME

The cortisol that your adrenal glands produce plays a role in the T4 to T3 conversion process. When cortisol levels are high, as when your adrenal glands increase cortisol production in response to stress, T4 to T3 conversion slows. This diverts the metabolic focus of your cells to generating the energy necessary for short-term response to a perceived crisis. Insulin sensitivity increases so your cells can burn more glucose, giving your body the burst of energy it needs to fight or flee. In this environment, T4 converts to rT3 instead of T3. The rT3 binds with cell and mitochondrial receptors. Because rT3 is significantly weaker than T3, this slows the cell's thyroid-hormone-driven processes.

There is speculation that when cortisol levels remain high over a long period of time rather than in the cyclical bursts of elevation that the stress-response matrix is designed to provide, the T4 to T3 conversion process becomes impaired. Even when cortisol levels return to normal (naturally or with treatment for adrenal fatigue), rT3 remains high. Short-term treatment with T3 supplement seems to restore the natural T4 to T3 conversion process.

There is speculation about the validity of rT3 dominance syndrome because as yet researchers can't directly observe the level of function that takes place within the thyroid receptors.

Improvements in technology and gains in understanding the role of DNA and gene structures in these kinds of functions might soon provide the scientific evidence doctors like to see before accepting such explanations. Whether or not rT3 "bumps" T3 from cell thyroid receptors, T3 supplementation does seem to improve symptoms related to underactive thyroid, especially when adrenal fatigue is also a factor.

Some people call rT3 dominance "Wilson's syndrome" after Dr. E. Denis Wilson, who described it. The treatment protocol in Wilson's syndrome usually involves "cycling" the body by using small doses of time-released T3 to raise the body temperature to normal ranges, then cycling down again. After two or three cycles, this protocol is said to reset the body's proper production of T3. Although there are no clinical studies to support or disprove this protocol, it is gaining interest as a treatment.

EUTHYROID SICK SYNDROME

Situations of severe trauma alter thyroid function without creating thyroid dysfunction. The resulting clinical picture is called euthyroid sick syndrome. Euthyroid sick syndrome is common with:

- Chronic illness
- Serious acute illness such as heart attack or stroke
- Major burns
- Malnutrition including starvation, fasting, and protein deprivation
- Major surgery
- Chronic kidney disease and failure
- Sepsis and shock

These are serious medical problems that require significant resources from your body. They are the kinds of stress your body's stress-response matrix is designed to handle, and altering thyroid function is one dimension of this response. It's not always easy to determine which is present, hypothyroidism or euthyroidism. Generally the laboratory findings with euthyroidism are:

- TSH levels are near normal
- T4 might be normal or slightly low
- T3 is low and rT3 is high
- T3 resin uptake is high

Treatment generally focuses on correcting the underlying health problems. Once those problems are under control, thyroid measurements often return to normal. If they don't, or if you have symptoms of thyroid imbalance, then underactive thyroid might also be a factor, and treating it would be appropriate.

9

The Autoimmune Connection

Your immune system protects your body from infections. Through a complex series of interactions, it identifies microorganisms and other substances as either friends or enemies. Friends can stay; enemies are attacked and, under ideal circumstances, eliminated. Many factors affect these processes, and sometimes they go awry. For reasons researchers don't fully understand, the body's defense mechanisms sometimes turn on certain cells within the body. Instead of attacking enemy invaders, your immune system can erroneously identify your own body tissues as alien and turn on them. These tissues can then no longer function properly, and the result is an autoimmune disorder. The kind of disorder depends on the tissues that are involved. An autoimmune response that targets the pancreas results in diabetes. An autoimmune response that targets cartilage and connective tissue results in rheumatoid arthritis. We believe that 90 percent or more of thyroid imbalance is autoimmune.

HOW YOUR IMMUNE RESPONSE FUNCTIONS

Your immune matrix, sometimes called your lymphatic system, consists of a network of structures that includes the following.

- Thymus gland
- Bone marrow
- Spleen
- Lymphocytes
- Lymph glands
- Lymphatic vessels
- Mucosa-associated lymph tissue (MALT)
- Gut-associated lymph tissue (GALT)

It also consists of a web of activities that involve other organs, tissues, cells, and functions throughout your body. There is a close interrelationship between your immunity matrix and your endocrine matrix.

THE THYMUS GLAND

The structure called the thymus is the "incubator" of your immune system. Its name comes from the Greek word *thymos*, meaning "warty"—a reference to its lobular, bumpy structure. This gland is located behind your breastbone, just below the level of your collarbones and over your heart. Its main purpose is to nurture immature T cells until they complete the complex molecular development process that makes them capable of functioning as the gatekeepers of your immune response. (More about T cells and the thymus gland's immune activities later in this chapter.)

The thymus develops early in the fetus, but doesn't become active until after birth. Throughout childhood and into early puberty, the thymus gland grows and produces the hormones that cause the lymphatic system to develop. Within the thymus, the cells that are to become your immune response grow to maturity. By adulthood the lymphatic system takes over responsibility for immune protection. After puberty, the thymus gland gradually decreases in both size and activity until it blends into the lymphatic system in the adult body. It also narrows to a single function: producing T cells, the "warriors" of your immune system. The thymus secretes a number of hormones, collectively known as thymic hormones. The main thymic hormones are:

- Thymosin
- Thymopoietin
- Thymulin
- Thymopentin
- Thymic humoral factor
- Thymostimulin

Although scientists have identified these hormones as distinct from one another, they don't know the exact functions of each. Overall, the thymic hormones appear to boost T-cell function. HIV/AIDS is bringing renewed focus to this connection. Some studies have shown improvement in symptoms and in the severity of disease in people with AIDS who took thymic hormone supplements. There are studies under way to examine whether thymic hormone supplements can reduce and even stop liver damage in people who have hepatitis C, a serious and potentially debilitating infection of the liver. Doctors sometimes give thymostimulin or thymic humoral factor supplement to boost the body's immune response to measles.

THE BONE MARROW

Bone marrow is a soft, pulpy substance in the center of most bones in the body. It contains stem cells, primitive structures that have the ability to develop into different kinds of blood cells depending on the hormone stimulation they receive. These are not the same stem cells that are attracting so much interest for their potential to grow into just about any kind of cell in the laboratory; those are embryonic stem cells. Because they exist at the early stages of life, embryonic stem cells appear to have virtually unlimited capacity to mature into cells of various tissues such as heart or lung or even thyroid. This potential may have far-reaching ramifications for future medical treatment options in many health conditions, although stem cell research is itself in what we might call an embryonic stage. Except for bone marrow transplant, stem cell therapy is still very experimental, and often controversial.

Stem cells in the adult body have far more limited capabilities and exist only in certain tissues, most prominently the bone marrow. Bone marrow stem cells can become erythrocytes (red blood cells), leukocytes (white blood cells), and platelets. Leukocytes are important in the body's immune response; these are the cells that attack, destroy, and literally consume invading "enemy" cells. There are numerous kinds of leukocytes, each with a specialized function. One is the lymphocyte, which is a key player in your immune response and in autoimmune disorders. Your spleen, lymph glands, and thymus gland also produce lymphocytes.

THE SPLEEN

Your spleen is a spongy, soft organ tucked just under the bottom of your ribs on your left side. It contains large amounts of lymph tissue, lymph cells, and lymphatic fluid. In an adult, the spleen has two primary functions:

- Destroy damaged, defective, and worn-out red blood cells
- Produce antibodies, phagocytes (white blood cells that consume invading microorganisms), and lymphocytes to fight infection

Blood flows through your spleen just as it flows through other filtering organs such as your liver and your kidneys. It passes through an intricate network of capillaries until finally it reaches the inner tissues of the spleen, called the red pulp. The lymph fluid that surrounds this network and bathes the red pulp is very dense with lymphocytes, and screens the blood for foreign microorganisms.

Even though these are important functions, other body systems can take them over if damage to your spleen means you must have surgery to remove it. Your spleen's extensive blood supply makes it very vulnerable to damage from blunt injury, such as from a forceful blow to the abdomen in a car accident or a fall. Other structures in your immune matrix then take over the spleen's functions. Your lymph glands, for example, similarly screen lymphatic fluid for microorganisms. If you no longer have your spleen, the lymphatic network intensifies its functions to help accommodate the loss.

THE LYMPHOCYTES

Lymphocytes are white blood cells that have extensive functions within your body's immune response. Like other white blood cells, they attack and consume invading microorganisms. They also program your immune response to recognize the same invaders if they return again, and to act against them to prevent them from starting an infection or illness. They do this by making proteins called antibodies or immunoglobulins. Your body makes millions of unique types of antibodies, each of which is sensitive to a specific microorganism. A small level of the antibody circulates in your bloodstream. If the substance to which it is sensitive enters your body, the antibody releases chemicals called cytokines that signal your body to produce more of the specific antibody. Antibodies serve to shield your body from invading microorganisms as well as attack those that make it through the antibody barrier. Immunizations (vaccines) also activate this response by intentionally introducing a weakened form of the microorganism into your body to stimulate an antibody response.

There are two general kinds of lymphocytes, T cells and B cells. Both originate in the bone marrow. Early in their development, T cells migrate to the thymus where they then come to maturity. B cells remain in the bone marrow, entering the bloodstream after maturing. Each has specific roles within your immune response.

Lymphocytes function rather like an army. T cells are the "special forces" that continually patrol your body via the lymph system and the circulatory system. When T cells encounter an invader, they send out chemical messages that muster the appropriate B cells. B cells then arrive to produce antibodies specific to the invading microorganism, tagging it as an enemy and preventing its advance into your body's systems.

SPECIAL FORCES: T CELLS

T cells, sometimes called T lymphocytes, have this name because they come to maturity in the thymus gland. There are three basic kinds of T cells: helper T cells, suppressor T cells, and cytotoxic (also called killer) T cells. Helper T cells identify, using complex chemical interactions, other cells that are bearers of infectious microorganisms such as bacteria or viruses. Suppressor T cells help to keep a lid on immune activity, preventing the incidental destruction of healthy body tissue. The balance between helper T cells, called T4 cells (not the same as the thyroid hormone T4), and suppressor T cells, called T8 cells, is the T-cell ratio. This ratio indicates whether the immune system is overfunctioning or underfunctioning. Cytotoxic T cells then respond to eliminate—kill—the contaminated cell. There are a number of subtypes of T cells that have specialized functions within this process.

TAKING CARE OF BUSINESS: B CELLS

B cells, sometimes called B lymphocytes, have this name because they come to maturity in the bone marrow. B cells produce and carry antibodies, and "remember" the microorganisms to which the antibodies are specific. When activated by the presence of a microorganism, B cells are capable of extremely rapid reproduction. Though they can't reproduce as fast as bacteria—a single bacterium can sometimes become a million bacteria in 8 to 12 hours—they can become a formidable reaction force within hours. The antibody response is very complex. Your body can have thousands (potentially millions) of kinds of different antibody-specific B cells.

LYMPH FLUID, VESSELS, AND NODES

Lymph fluid is similar to blood except that it doesn't contain any red blood cells, so rather than being red it is very pale, almost like watery milk. It carries leukocytes (white blood cells) and substances with molecules too large to travel through the blood vessels, such as some proteins. About 20 to 30 percent of the leukocytes in lymph fluid are lymphocytes, primarily T cells and B cells. At any given time your body contains about three quarts of lymph, which it circulates, uses, and replenishes every 24 hours.

Lymph travels through a network similar in structure to your network of blood vessels. The lymph vessels run alongside your major blood vessels. As it travels through this network, lymph collects and carries along a variety of waste products, toxins, and other cellular debris. It passes its collection into your bloodstream, and your blood transports it to your liver and kidneys, which filter it and excrete it along with all the other waste products in your blood.

The major lymph vessel is the thoracic duct; it parallels your aorta along the length of your chest and abdomen. Unlike your circulatory system, your lymph network has no heart or other pumping mechanism to move fluid through it. It relies instead on gravity and on the gentle massaging action of your muscles during activity. During long periods of inactivity, such as during extended illness, lymph flow slows. Extended inactivity can make your immune response less effective.

Lymph glands are not really glands but rather are nodes of tissue along the lymph vessels. They store lymphocytes and other leukocytes. You have lymph nodes all along the lymph vessels throughout your body, around six hundred of them. The only ones you usually notice are the ones that occur in clusters near the surface of your skin, such as those under your arm (axillary lymph nodes), in your groin (inguinal lymph nodes), and in your neck (cervical lymph nodes). When there is an infection in your body, those cells (primarily B cells) in the lymph nodes closest to the site of the infection multiply rapidly. This causes the lymph node to swell; it can't dump the cells out into your lymph fluid fast enough to keep pace with their reproduction.

Lymph nodes also contain "eater" cells called macrophages; they consume microorganisms and cells that cytotoxic T cells attack and destroy. This activity causes further swelling during infection, as the macrophages become engorged. Eventually the lymph node discharges its contents—lymphocytes and macrophagic waste—into the lymph for transport into the bloodstream. The lymphocytes swarm into action to fight your infection, and your blood carries the waste on to the filtering mechanisms that will remove it from your body.

It's an amazingly complex and efficient system, although not foolproof. Infections and diseases can overwhelm your immune response. Some viruses, such as the deadly Ebola virus, mask themselves so well that by the time your T cells identify them as invaders it's too late for their attack to overcome the infection.

Cancer also can overpower your immune response. There is some evidence, in fact, that B cells themselves become mutated into cancerous cells to cause certain lymphomas (cancers of the lymph structures). And your immune response can turn on healthy, normal cells within your body, treating them as invaders. This disables or destroys their functions, creating a disease condition—an autoimmune disorder—that originates from within your body rather than attacking it from outside.

MUCOSA-ASSOCIATED LYMPH TISSUE (MALT) AND GUT-ASSOCIATED LYMPH TISSUE (GALT)

Mucosa-associated lymph tissue (MALT) exists throughout your body in tissues that have mucous membranes, such as in your urinary tract. Gut-associated lymph tissue (GALT) exists in your intestinal tract. These tissues are extensions of the lymph system and have heightened immune activity. Tonsils and adenoids are probably the most familiar GALTs. These structures, located at the back of your mouth and at the top of your throat, frequently swell when you have a viral infection such as a cold or the flu. This swelling is often painful, and the lymph tissues themselves can become infected.

YOUR THYMUS GLAND AND YOUR IMMUNE RESPONSE

Until the 1960s, doctors believed the thymus gland was ordinarily small and then swelled in response to illness or infection. They drew this conclusion from the only information that was available to them about the thymus gland: autopsy results. Coroners noticed that babies who died without explanation, such as a result of sudden infant death syndrome (SIDS), had enormously large thymus glands, while children who died from infection and disease had very small thymus glands. There was even a name for this "disease"—status thymicolymphaticus or status thymicus. It often became the cause of death when no other cause was obvious and the thymus was large enough to be detectable.

PAST MISUNDERSTANDINGS, CURRENT CONSEQUENCES

In the 1940s, 1950s, and early 1960s, a common treatment for "enlarged" thymus was radiation. Doctors ordered the treatment in the mistaken belief that an enlarged thymus would cause potentially life-threatening disease. Prevailing medical wisdom held that forcing the thymus to shrink would subsequently eliminate its ability to cause illness and prevent the nearly always fatal status thymicolymphaticus. It appeared to be a successful treatment because those who had it done seemed to avoid serious illness afterward. But appearances aren't always what they seem. Children outgrow the propensity for certain diseases, inherently reducing their risk. What appeared to be a consequence of medical intervention was in fact nothing more than a function of nature.

We now know that these were erroneous conclusions drawn from observations that preceded our understanding of how the thymus gland functions. We now know that the thymus is not only proportionately larger in children, but also begins growing shortly following birth and continues to grow until about age 14. At its peak size, the thymus gland is large enough to cover the outside of the heart. And we now know that the thymus gland, because of its role in the immune system, shrinks during times of stress and when an infection is present, when the body calls on the T cells that it manufactures. When demand depletes supply, the thymus shrinks and stays small until it rebuilds its stock of T cells.

Unfortunately, medical intervention to shrink the thymus had several unexpected and undesirable side effects. Many people who underwent radiation treatment for "enlarged" thymus now have immune response problems including various autoimmune disorders. And many of them have hypothyroidism, a combined result of autoimmune activity and radiation damage to the thyroid gland. Forty years ago radiation treatment was not nearly as precise as it is today, and radiation beams were wide enough to contact a wide circle of surrounding tissues. Radiation aimed at the thymus gland also struck the thyroid gland. Its sensitive tissues withered and died under the attack, and thyroid function diminished or even ended.

THE THYMUS-AUTOIMMUNE CONNECTION

When doctors began to understand the functions of the various lymphatic cells (lymphocytes) and the thymus gland's role in bringing T cells to maturity, it became clear that the thymus has an integral connection to autoimmune activity as well as immune function. Doctors are exploring this connection as a path to treatment for certain autoimmune conditions. One is myasthenia gravis, in which the body's immune response attacks acetylcholine receptors in voluntary muscle cells.

Acetylcholine is a chemical that functions as a neurotransmitter; that is, it facilitates communication between nerve cells and other cells. Acetylcholine reaches out from the nerve cell to the muscle cell. If it finds an open receptor, it binds. This permits the nerve cell to send signals to the muscle cell; these signals result in movement. When there is a disruption of this process, communication between nerve cells and muscle cells becomes erratic. Even though both kinds of cells (and the tissues they form) are normal, the connection between them is distorted. The result is poor muscle contraction and muscle weakness that can be debilitating, especially when it affects the muscles of the throat (affecting swallowing) and chest (affecting breathing).

Doctors have noticed that people with myasthenia gravis often have enlarged thymus glands and some even have tumors (usually benign, or noncancerous) of the thymus. This suggests a connection between the condition and T-cell maturation.

One theory is that something goes awry with T-cell programming that instructs T cells to read the proteins of acetylcholine receptors as antigens, or enemy invaders. Surgically removing the thymus markedly improves myasthenia gravis symptoms in many people who have the condition.

Such surgery is a major undertaking, however. The thymus lies behind the sternum (breastbone), making access difficult—the surgeon must cut through this thick, protective bone. Full recovery is about the same as for open-heart surgery—four to six weeks for most people. This makes this surgery, called thymectomy, a treatment to consider only after other treatments have failed. And it doesn't make thymectomy particularly inviting as an experimental treatment for other autoimmune disorders.

LYMPHOCYTES AND AUTOIMMUNE RESPONSE

When there is an autoimmune response affecting an organ or body system, a biopsy of the affected tissue generally shows infiltration with lymph fluid and cells—far more than is present when the tissue is healthy. T cells and B cells have rallied to the attack, destroying the tissue they've now identified as the enemy. This interferes with the structure's function. In the case of endocrine glands such as the pancreas or thyroid, the result can be complete shutdown of the gland's function.

One theory is that, as with myasthenia gravis, such responses originate with "programming" errors of the T cells that occur in the thymus. Defective T cells emerge from the thymus ready to identify certain body tissues as "enemy" even though they're not. Another theory is that the B cells make the mistake, producing antibodies that attack body proteins as though they were antigens. In either case, the immune response turns on the tissues that it should be protecting.

Researchers don't fully understand how an autoimmune response develops, but they do know that once there is one at work in your body there are likely to be others. This points the finger of suspicion at the thymus and its role in bringing T cells to maturation, because T cells are responsible for identifying both normal cells and invading microorganisms. It is likely that there is an interaction of some sort between such programming malfunctions and genetic encoding, although this connection is not conclusive.

AUTOIMMUNE RESPONSE AND THE ENDOCRINE MATRIX

When autoimmune response attacks an endocrine structure, the first reaction is inflammation and swelling. Most of the time you don't notice this because the structure is deep within your body. One exception is the thyroid gland, which is very near the skin surface. Swelling in the thyroid produces the familiar symptom of goiter. The two most common thyroid conditions, Hashimoto's thyroiditis and Graves' disease, we know to be autoimmune disorders. We suspect that nearly all thyroid imbalance is also autoimmune in origin.

When one endocrine structure becomes the target of an autoimmune attack, it is likely, although not certain, that other structures will also become involved. We don't know yet whether this is because endocrine cells are similar enough that T cells expand their erroneous identification to them as invaders or because the imbalance in one endocrine structure stresses other endocrine structures to create weaknesses that make their tissues vulnerable. It's possible that very subtle changes take place in failing endocrine tissues that cause them to appear foreign to the T cells. As yet, however, the intricate mechanisms involved have evaded researchers.

AUTOIMMUNE TRIGGERS

It appears that there are a number of triggers that can activate an autoimmune response, which suggests that continued stress (of any kind) to the immune matrix weakens its ability to function. Researchers believe external factors like environmental toxins trigger immune overreactions in some cases. Allergies, particularly food allergies, are implicated in the development of autoimmune illnesses. Chronic infections also may activate the immune system, leading to the creation of autoantibodies. Autoimmune diseases such as rheumatoid arthritis and ulcerative colitis seem to have infectious origins.

Long-term physical and emotional stress can produce interleukins and other immune proteins that can activate the immune system. It's possible, although not proven, that one reason women are more affected than men by autoimmune disorders has to do with the continuous cycling of hormones in their bodies. An imbalance in one part of the endocrine matrix, however slight and even if not functionally perceptible, affects the balance and function of all parts.

BOOSTING IMMUNE FUNCTION TO IMPROVE THYROID BALANCE

It makes sense that doing what you can to keep your immune matrix functioning at peak performance is a benefit to all structures and systems of your body—to your overall health. The most effective ways to do this are amazingly simple:

- Drink plenty of water, at least 8 to 12 full glasses daily. You really can't drink too much water, and most people drink far too little.
- Get adequate sleep. For most people, this is seven to nine hours of uninterrupted sleep *at night*. Remember, the

cortisol cycle that supports your body's health follows the circadian cycle of darkness and light. In addition, a hormone called melatonin, produced by the pineal gland, rises at night, and has a profound effect on the immune system, resetting it for the next day. People who work shifts and sleep during daylight hours often have more illness because these cycles become imbalanced.

- Eat nutritiously. Your body needs the raw materials that a balanced diet provides, so it can build healthy cells and tissues.

- If you have an autoimmune illness, consider searching for food allergies. You can do this by withdrawing the most common food allergens for a minimum of five days, and then adding them back one by one. Many times, symptoms will get better when certain foods are withdrawn, and return when those foods are added back. The most common food allergens are wheat, yeast, dairy, eggs, citrus, coffee, corn, and soy.

- Stay active. Physical activity keeps lymph flowing, which maximizes its ability to stop infections before you notice any ill effects. Physical activity, especially moderate to intense exercise on a regular basis, is key to the health of many body systems and indeed your overall health (more on this in later chapters).

If you are at particular risk for autoimmune disorders, either because you already have at least one (such as thyroid imbalance) or because you have stressors in your life that you can't eliminate (such as shift work), you might want to boost your immune response through dietary supplements such as zinc, vitamin C, and folic acid, and herbs such as garlic and milk thistle.

Several studies support the use of essential fatty acids, particularly fish oils, in autoimmune diseases such as rheumatoid arthritis, systemic lupus erythematosis, and psoriasis. Flax oil also seems to have positive effects, perhaps because it contains lignans, natural chemicals that improve the immune barrier of the gut.

Garlic, berberine, and olive leaf all have immune-strengthening activity. Echinacea does as well, but may stimulate the immune system too much; doctors of natural medicine generally suggest avoiding or limiting echinacea when there is autoimmune illness. Milk thistle is an herb that helps the liver break down the waste products of the immune system, and is useful with autoimmune diseases. Rhodiola and Eleutherococcus (Siberian ginseng) can help to cushion the body against stresses.

Recently, an extract of colostrum, the immune-enhancing liquid secreted before breast milk comes in, has been used to balance the overactivity of the immune system in autoimmune illness. This extract contains transfer factors, proteins that have been studied for their controlling effects on immune cells. Finally, there is some suggestion that thymus extracts and supplements may have some role in treating autoimmune diseases.

Part 3

Thyroid Therapies

10

Treatment Approaches for Underactive Thyroid

If your doctor has diagnosed hypothyroidism, you're probably taking a daily thyroid hormone supplement. And odds are, you're going to take it for the rest of your life. The goal of hormone supplementation is to restore your thyroid balance as close as possible to its natural level. A number of products are available for doctors to prescribe for this purpose. They fall into two main categories, synthetic and natural.

There is considerable debate as to whether one form is better than the other, and whether T4 supplementation alone is adequate or whether you also need T3 supplementation. Doctors and people with underactive thyroid all have their preferences. In the end, however, what matters most is what works for *you*. And what is most important is knowing all of the options that are available to you, and their advantages and disadvantages, so you can make informed decisions about *your* treatment approach.

There are also numerous nonpharmaceutical therapies used to boost underactive thyroid. Some of these are helpful when your blood thyroid-hormone levels are technically "normal"—that is, when you do not have clinical hypothy-roidism as conventional medicine defines it but you have symp-toms of underactive thyroid. Some may or may not be helpful, but are not likely to be harmful. And there are some that are potentially dangerous.

No substance that you put into your body is without risk, whether or not you need a doctor's prescription to take it, and combining products can have unexpected results. Always use cau-tion! Hypothyroidism affects every system in your body, and if left untreated has serious health consequences (with the rare com-plication of myxedemic coma being potentially fatal). Although your health is ultimately in your hands, it's a good idea to stay in close contact with your regular health-care practitioner if you are diagnosed hypothyroid, have symptoms of underactive thyroid, or are taking any products to boost thyroid balance. Chapter 12 discusses how to make choices and decisions about treatment to create your personal approach for thyroid balance.

SYNTHETIC T4 SUPPLEMENTS

In the United States, the current standard of treatment—the point at which many doctors start in their attempts to bring your thyroid back into balance—for hypothyroidism is synthetic T4 supplementation. Synthetic T4 supplement drugs contain the thyroid hormone levothyroxine (also called l-thyroxine), derived from synthetic sources—made in a laboratory. Chemically, synthetic levothyroxine is identical to the thyroxine (T4) your thyroid gland produces.

The brand-name version of this drug, Synthroid, was the first synthetic thyroid hormone product to be developed, and has had a strong hold on the market since its introduction in the early 1960s. According to its manufacturer, more than eight mil-lion people worldwide take Synthroid daily. Synthroid has become synonymous with thyroid treatment, and people often use the brand name to refer broadly to all synthetic levothyroxine products.

AVAILABLE LEVOTHYROXINE PRODUCTS

There are four levothyroxine products available in the United States today:

- Levothroid
- Levoxyl
- Synthroid
- Unithroid

All but Synthroid are generic formulas; they came onto the market after the patent on Synthroid expired, making it legal to make competitive products. Because every manufacturer uses different inactive ingredients in compounding their thyroid tablets, doctors and pharmacists generally recommend that once you start taking a particular brand you stay with that brand. Changing among brands can lead to inconsistent thyroid hormone levels with each new prescription.

A study reported in the *New England Journal of Medicine* in 1999 challenged this long-standing perception. It concluded that despite minor variations in blood levels, all brands of levothyroxine currently available in the United States are generally bioequivalent—that is, they all deliver the same amount of levothyroxine per dosage strength. The variations that do occur, the study determined, arise from differences in absorption (how easily the drug gets from your digestive system into your bloodstream) and other differences in the ways people take their thyroid hormone supplements.

Rather than resolving the questions about bioequivalency across brands, the study fueled the debate. Most doctors and pharmacists continue to recommend that you stay with the brand that seems to relieve your symptoms. Your body's response to thyroid hormone is very sensitive, whether that hormone comes from within your body or you take it as a supplement. How much hormone you get from each pill must be consistent within a very narrow margin. Technically, this is known as a narrow therapeutic index.

This doesn't mean you're stuck with the first brand of levothyroxine that you try. Some people have better success with one brand over another, for any number of reasons. It's possible to react to the filler ingredients, or to find that one brand absorbs into your system faster or more consistently than another. You might want to switch to a generic product to save money. Whatever your reason, always remember it is your choice. Just ask your doctor to check your blood thyroid hormone levels just as if you were first starting on the medication. This way, you'll know whether there are any differences and also you'll be sure you're getting the appropriate dose. It's possible that your doctor might need to adjust your dose after you switch brands.

THE LEVOTHYROXINE CONTROVERSY

Despite its reign as the standard of treatment for hypothyroidism for decades, levothyroxine became embroiled in controversy in the late 1990s when Synthroid and other synthetic levothyroxine preparations came under scrutiny from the United States Food and Drug Administration (FDA). This was largely in response to complaints from patients and doctors about apparent potency inconsistencies among products and even within product lines. People noticed they felt different from one prescription to another, raising suspicion that potency varied from one manufacturing batch to another.

Indeed, this turned out to be the case. In 1997, the FDA ordered all manufacturers of synthetic thyroid supplement to conduct tests to determine their product line's potency, stability, and bioavailability (amount of drug that actually makes it into circulation after you take the drug). To virtually no one's surprise, the tests demonstrated inconsistencies. Synthroid, the first levothyroxine product on the market, was available before there were regulations requiring drugs to be approved before they could be sold. When the FDA and its regulations came into effect, Synthroid, along with hundreds of other drugs already being sold, were grandfathered into an approval status without being required to go through the approval process.

No two batches of anything can ever be absolutely identical, of course. Minor variations are typical and generally without consequence. But the testing the FDA ordered confirmed that levothyroxine formulas varied too widely and were unacceptably inconsistent. The FDA ordered manufacturers to reformulate their products, and, for the first time, submit them to the FDA for approval as new drugs. By summer 2002, all levothyroxine products currently on the market had received approval.

IS LEVOTHYROXINE FOR YOU?

The majority of people who take levothyroxine for underactive thyroid find that it relieves most of their symptoms most of the time. Many people find that it relieves their symptoms all of the time. And some people find that it makes little or no difference in how they feel, even if their blood thyroid levels return to normal. If you're taking levothyroxine and you feel fine and your blood thyroid levels are normal, then levothyroxine is a good choice for you. If you continue to have symptoms of underactive thyroid, you might want to explore other treatment approaches.

The key advantages to taking levothyroxine are that it is readily available, is reasonably priced (especially generic formulas), and comes in up to eleven strengths to make it easier to find the dose that works for you. When you first start taking levothyroxine, your doctor will order blood tests to measure its effectiveness. Generally these are scheduled for one, three, and six months after your treatment begins. If your test results are within normal ranges at the six-month point, your doctor will suggest annual rechecks to make sure your thyroid balance remains stable.

HOW MUCH LEVOTHYROXINE SHOULD YOU TAKE?

Levothyroxine strength is usually expressed in micrograms—for example, 25 mcg. If expressed in milligrams, this same strength would be written as 0.25 mg. Levothyroxine products are available in incremental strengths starting at 25 mcg and extending to 300 mcg. Not all products include the entire range; some stop at an upper strength of 200 mcg. There really is no set starting point for dosing. Doctors tend to start with a fairly low dose, such as 25 mcg or 50 mcg, and see what happens. Ten people with very similar blood-test results are likely to have ten entirely different responses to the same dose, so finding the dose that works for you probably will be a process of trial and error.

Changes in your health, lifestyle, and even just age can change the effectiveness of your levothyroxine dose. Gaining or losing a significant amount of weight, developing chronic health problems, becoming more or less physically active, experiencing changes in stress, even changing the way you eat—all of these factors influence how your body absorbs and uses thyroid hormone. This is why doctors recommend annual blood tests to measure your thyroid hormone levels. Test results, of course, are not the definitive answer as to whether or not a treatment is succeeding. You need to keep track of how you feel so you can report any changes in your symptoms to your doctor. Chapter 12 discusses ways to find and maintain the treatment balance that works best for you.

NATURAL DESICCATED T4 SUPPLEMENTS

Doctors have been treating underactive thyroid with some form of hormone supplementation for about two hundred years.

When hormone treatment began, supplements came from dried, pulverized, and purified thyroid tissues extracted from animals, usually cows and sometimes sheep. The thyroid glands were harvested during slaughter and shipped to laboratories that then prepared the tissue and compounded it into tablets. The result was called desiccated thyroid extract.

The primary challenge of this process was trying to make the tablets of uniform potency. The amount of thyroxine extracted from each cow's thyroid gland varied, of course, because the amount of thyroxine the thyroid glands contained varied from animal to animal. The typical means of measuring the powdered extract was by weight or volume, neither of which accounted for concentration of thyroxine. As well, the thyroid glands contained other thyroid hormones, primarily T3. This made dosing even trickier. Not only were the concentrations of both T4 and the more potent T3 unknown, but the ratio between the two hormones was a mystery, too. In short, you never really knew what you were taking.

Crowning these challenges was the factor of cost. Harvesting, preparing, and compounding the thyroid glands of animals was a very time-consuming and expensive process. These inconsistencies led to the development of Synthroid, which was the first synthetic form of thyroxine. After Synthroid gained acceptance, natural desiccated thyroid fell out of favor. The original formulation from cow thyroid is no longer available in the United States, primarily because of the threat that it could be contaminated with the infectious agent that causes bovine spongiform encephalopathy (BSE), the so-called "mad cow disease."

TODAY'S NATURAL DESICCATED THYROID PRODUCTS

Natural desiccated thyroid products available on the market today are derived from pig, or porcine, thyroids. Porcine thyroid tissue is easier to obtain and does not carry the potential risk of BSE and related animal diseases that can cause infection in humans. As well, modern manufacturing practices made purification more complete. Dosing is also more consistent, although it still varies more than with synthetic products. There are also nonpharmaceutical products that contain weak mixtures of desiccated thyroid, sold as dietary supplements. More on these later in this chapter.

Products containing natural desiccated thyroid hormone extract that currently are available include:

- Armour Thyroid
- Nature-Thyroid
- Thyroid USP
- Westhyroid

These products are all considered bioequivalent; that is, each product delivers the same potency of thyroid hormone per dose. In addition to T4, these products contain traces of T3, T2, and other hormonal substances found naturally in thyroid tissue. People who support natural over synthetic supplements view this as an advantage because it's virtually impossible to replicate all of these substances in the laboratory. We don't know precisely what their functions are or how they affect one another, drawing some people to conclude that even so they must serve some useful purpose or they wouldn't be present in nature. Even though natural desiccated thyroid products contain trace amounts of T3, they are not considered T4-T3 combination products. The measurement is of the amount of T4.

Is Natural Desiccated Thyroid the Choice for You?

People who continue to have symptoms of underactive thyroid after trying levothyroxine for a period of time (six months is a good minimum) sometimes find that switching to a natural desiccated thyroid supplement relieves their symptoms. This is probably because of the trace amounts of T3 and other hormonal substances that natural desiccated products contain, although there is little scientific evidence to support this perception. If natural desiccated thyroid relieves your symptoms when levothyroxine has not, however, scientific evidence means very little! Doctors with a holistic or integrative approach to health and health care often choose a natural desiccated thyroid product when starting new treatment for underactive thyroid.

NATURAL DESICCATED THYROID STRENGTHS AND DOSING

The strength of natural desiccated thyroid products is measured in milligrams and generally starts at 15 mg. Sometimes you'll see the old-fashioned "grain" measurement; 15 mg is roughly equivalent to 1/4 grain, and a full 1 grain strength is equivalent to 60 mg. There really isn't a standard starting point for dosing; doctors typically start with a fairly low dose and build up to the dose that relieves your symptoms without causing other problems. Expect regular blood tests until your thyroid levels stabilize, and then blood tests annually.

T3 SUPPLEMENTATION: IS T4 ALONE ENOUGH?

If your thyroid produces, and your body uses, T3, doesn't it make sense to supplement or replace it as well when thyroid function is low? This practical question has a convoluted, and in the end inconclusive, answer. Remember, T3 is many times more potent than T4, and affects cells almost immediately. This makes the potential for overdose quite high. Your body accommodates this sensitivity by having just a limited amount of T3 in circulation, even though it's T3 that your cells must have. Your body makes T3 by converting it from T4, a time-consuming process. If the demand for T3 exceeds the rate of conversion, your endocrine matrix can then boost T3 production in your thyroid gland to get the T3 out there right away. As further proof of the marvelous interconnectedness of body processes, varied factors affect the conversion to T3 including stress; amount of saturated fat in the diet; various nutrients, herbs and medications; and even exercise. In any case, the process is complex enough that when your thyroid is in balance, it's very unlikely that you'll have too much T3 circulating in your system.

That's not the case when you take a T3 supplement. The amount you take goes immediately into your bloodstream. If you take too much, you can experience temporary symptoms of hyperthyroidism: jitters, rapid pulse, feelings of nervousness. It's this narrow margin of safety that makes doctors uneasy about prescribing T3. Some doctors try to get around it by having a pharmacy compound a time-release formula. This treatment works very well in some people, but it is time-consuming and expensive, and not all pharmacies are capable of doing it. Taking a tyrosine dietary supplement along with a T3 supplement seems to smooth out the T3 effect and response for some people (see Chapter 15 for more about nutrition and thyroid function). If you're taking a T3 supplement, be very vigilant about how you feel. Contact your doctor right away if you begin to experience any symptoms that might suggest overactive thyroid (resulting from too much T3 supplement). The symptoms generally pass within six to eight hours since the active life of T3 is so short.

Most often, your doctor will prescribe T3 in combination with T4. This helps to offset the potential problems of T3 supplementation alone. Sometimes doctors will prescribe T3 alone if you are preparing for a thyroid scan and have to be off your T4 supplement. The T3 will keep the symptoms of underactive thyroid at bay, but doesn't stay in your body long enough to alter thyroid function. The brand name of T3 available in the

United States is Cytomel, which contains liothyronine. Liothyronine is a synthetic (laboratory-created) form of tri-iodothyronine (T3).

Some doctors are using Cytomel in very small doses to treat a variety of symptoms, including hair loss (alopecia), fatigue, and depression. These doses, around 5 mcg daily, are not high enough to suppress the body's own thyroid function, and usually do not cause problems associated with larger amounts of T3.

COMBINATION T4-T3 SUPPLEMENTS

Supplement products relatively new to the market are those that combine T4 and T3 in the same pill. The main advantage of this is that you only have to take one pill to get two drugs. The drawback is that it's far more challenging to find the right balance of doses. You might get a combination that has the right amount of T4 for you, but too little or too much T3 . . . or the reverse. Because T3 is so much more potent than T4, it is more often the component that is difficult to dose.

If you already take T4 and T3 but in separate pills and you know which strengths work best for you, you might find it more convenient to switch to a combination product that offers the same respective strengths. For most people, taking T4 and T3 separately is a better choice. The combination product available in the United States is Liotrix, sold under the brand name Thyrolar. It is a synthetic product, a combination of liothyronine and levothyroxine.

TAKING THYROID SUPPLEMENT CORRECTLY

One factor that contributes significantly to variations in the effectiveness of thyroid hormone supplements, whether in natural or synthetic forms, is inconsistency in the way they're taken. Variations in timing by as little as an hour, and in the kinds of foods you eat and how much time passes between eating them and taking your thyroid supplement, add up to make big differences in how rapidly the hormone is absorbed into your bloodstream and how much of it actually makes it into your body. Be sure to follow these guidelines:

- Take your thyroid supplement at the same time each day, and take it every day.
- Take your thyroid supplement one hour before or two hours after eating, so you take it on an empty stomach. Food can affect how much thyroid hormone gets absorbed into your system.
- If you are taking thyroid supplement, do not take other medications, prescription or over-the-counter, without talking to your doctor or pharmacist.
- Check refilled prescriptions to make sure you receive the same brand of thyroid hormone that you've been taking.
- Do not take your thyroid supplement at the same time you take vitamins, iron, calcium, or other dietary supplements. These products interfere with how thyroid hormone gets into your system.

Consistency is key. Get settled into a routine for taking your thyroid medication, and then stick with it. This makes it easier to evaluate your situation if the hormone supplement doesn't relieve your symptoms, and makes it easier for you to identify any changes or problems as they might arise.

NONPHARMACEUTICAL THERAPIES

Through the centuries of human existence, there have been many ways to treat thyroid imbalance. These include substances such as kelp (seaweed) and dulse (another kind of seaweed), as well as certain herbs and dietary supplements. For underactive thyroid in which lab test results support a hypothyroidism diagnosis, nonpharmaceutical therapies won't be sufficient to give your body the thyroid hormones it needs. In such a case, relying solely on these therapies is probably going to create health problems for you, some of which are potentially life-threatening. You might choose to include them in your personal plan for achieving thyroid balance, however, as we discuss in later chapters.

NUTRITIONAL REMEDIES

It seems natural to look to nutrition as a therapy for thyroid imbalance. Many foods contain elements, such as iodine, that are essential for healthy thyroid function. Substances such as tyrosine, an amino acid your thyroid gland requires to make T4 and T3 from iodine, are found in many foods as well. Kelp and dulse, kinds of seaweed that are high in iodine, are other nutritional substances that can aid thyroid function. The herb bladder wrack is also high in iodine.

Some dietary supplements actually contain weak forms of thyroid hormones. Thyroid glandular is a mild preparation of desiccated thyroid extract sold in the United States as a dietary supplement, for example, and used in naturopathic and other treatments. Chapter 15 discusses nutrition and thyroid balance in detail.

HOMEOPATHIC REMEDIES

Homeopathy, developed in Europe in the eighteenth century, is a very different way of using medicines to treat illness. The "Law of Similars," upon which homeopathy is based, says that if a substance (herb, mineral, organism) causes certain symptoms or disease, then giving a very dilute form of that substance can coax the body to heal those symptoms or disease. It's similar to the conventional medicine concept of vaccination, where tiny amounts of a weakened organism are used to stimulate immunity in the body toward that organism in its strong form. For a homeopath, very dilute forms of iodine might be used to treat hyperthyroidism and symptoms of iodine poisoning.

The dilutions, however, are what make homeopathy so controversial. Homeopathic formulations are diluted so much that it becomes highly improbable that there are any molecules of the substance left in the remedy! It's as if a picture of a doctor were used to treat a patient. The energetic memory of the substance is kept in the diluting water and, when given to the person, allows healing to take place. This provides a second law of homeopathy, that the body has an innate drive toward healing and balance, and just has to be reminded of this.

Although the science behind homeopathy is yet to be proved satisfactorily, there is no question that the world medical literature contains several well-constructed studies demonstrating its positive effects. And, over half the world's population uses homeopathy as part of their medical care. Since thyroid problems can be caused by a variety of factors, a classical homeopath (who uses a single remedy to treat the patient) might draw from a variety of substances. Other homeopaths use a variety of remedies together to treat metabolic problems, including very dilute forms of thyroid itself. Homeopathy is a very safe form of medicine. Many homeopaths prefer that a patient is off other natural treatments, but it's not likely that they will, nor is it safe to, go off thyroid medication while waiting for a homeopathic remedy to take effect.

THE TRADITIONAL CHINESE MEDICINE (TCM) PERSPECTIVE

The Western view of thyroid balance and imbalance is rooted in the analysis of body systems and how they function both independently and interrelatedly. The emphasis is on hormone excess and deficiency. In the Eastern view, thyroid balance and imbalance are simply pieces of a bigger balance and imbalance picture: yin and yang. These are the two bookends of existence, representing opposite characteristics that then blend into a balanced whole. In life, these two principles are constantly changing into the other, rising, falling, and rising again much like day and night or summer and winter. Just as the hormonal metabolic matrix consists of many organs that we can't fully understand without looking at their relationship to the whole, so yin and yang are not separate principles; each exists within a dynamic relationship to the other.

Yin is darker, moist, colder, receptive, and feminine. Yang is lighter, dry, hotter, giving, and masculine. Health is a matter of balancing yin and yang. It also is a matter of balancing qi, or life energy, and the flow of qi through the body's energy systems. Imbalance results from impeded flow; restoring balance restores the flow of qi. For Westerners who have trouble with this concept, think of qi as the equivalent of, or comparable to, the flow of information from the body's hormonal matrixes that promotes balance throughout the body's systems.

From the Eastern perspective, underactive thyroid results from an imbalance in which yin dominates and yang is deficient, since there is less activity and less heat. TCM uses herbal preparations to bring the yin-yang balance back into alignment. Common remedies for underactive thyroid are kidney yang tonic (jin gui hen qi wan) and right restoration formula (tou gui wan). These remedies are available through TCM practitioners.

There are many styles of acupuncture practiced in the United States currently. Chinese (TCM), Japanese, Five Element, and French Energetics styles of acupuncture share in common the use of needles in points called acu-points, found along channels called meridians that traverse the body. The needles encourage the flow of "qi," the Chinese word for the life force that circulates through the body in the meridians and into the organs. Thyroid problems, like any other illness, are treated with acupuncture according to the diagnosis of that system. Generally, because the thyroid is involved with temperature regulation, a meridian called the Triple Warmer is involved, and frequently another channel called the Pericardium, or Circulation-Sex channel.

Interestingly, there are some Western studies of acupuncture that involve the thyroid gland. For instance, some research has shown that acu-point stimulation releases TSH, along with ACTH and other pituitary hormones.

THYROID SUPPLEMENTATION WHEN LAB RESULTS ARE "NORMAL"

"Normal" is one of those subjective, shifting definitions. It changes in relationship to its context. It also applies across a broad spectrum, with the recognition that at either end of that spectrum what's normal in one person might be a clinical problem in another. Because we all like definitions that are clean and precise, however, we've come to identify "normal" as an absolute.

In January 2001, the American Association of Clinical Endocrinologists made the startling, though long overdue, shift in perspective to recommend that doctors consider treating people whose TSH levels are between 3.0 and 5.5, even though that is within the range of "normal" levels. This reflects a growing awareness within conventional medicine that thyroid balance is a far more narrow range than previously thought. It also broadens the scope of "treatable" thyroid imbalance to include people whose primary indication of thyroid imbalance is symptom-based rather than lab-based, and improves the possibility that, in the near future, thyroid function will be judged within the context of the entire metabolic matrix.

11

Treatment Approaches for Overactive Thyroid

Treatment for overactive thyroid, or hyperthyroidism, aims to slow thyroid hormone production. There are two basic ways to accomplish this goal: drugs (including radioactive iodine therapy) and surgery. For most people, drugs are the first treatment of choice. Drugs are less invasive, and are successful in permanently returning your thyroid gland to normal function about half the time.

Of course, this means they are *not* effective about half the time. When this is the case, surgery becomes the only alternative for slowing thyroid activity. Because most hyperthyroidism appears suddenly (even if it has been building for some time), its symptoms are dramatic and uncomfortable, and its potential health dangers are serious (such as heart irregularities and damage to the optic nerves), so treatment usually begins promptly.

ANTITHYROID DRUGS

The drugs that slow thyroid function are called antithyroid drugs. The different drugs have somewhat different processes, but the end result is the same: they end a certain amount of thyroid hormone production. Some, such as radioactive iodine, accomplish this by killing off hormone-producing cells in the thyroid gland, reducing the gland's capability to produce T3 and T4. Others target the T4-to-T3 conversion process, creating interference that inhibits or slows it.

RADIOACTIVE IODINE THERAPY

Radioactive iodine therapy, or I^{131}, is sometimes called a chemical thyroidectomy. This treatment effectively destroys thyroid tissue, rendering it incapable of producing thyroid hormones. This is the same result as if the tissue were surgically removed, but without the invasion of surgery. As with surgery, the outcome is somewhat unpredictable. Some people become hypothyroid within a year or two, and then must receive treatment for that.

Doctors use the results of a radioactive iodine uptake test combined with a scan to determine the dose of I^{131} that you need. They then mix this dose into a powdered preparation that fits into a standard medicine capsule. You swallow the capsule, and the I^{131} is absorbed into your system through your digestive tract. You won't taste or feel anything when you take the capsule, and won't notice any effect for about six weeks. It can take three to six months to see the full effect.

This treatment approach came into existence in 1946, when doctors realized that people who had been exposed to high levels of radiation during tests of atomic bombs (and in the use of atomic bombs to end World War II) experienced significant thyroid dysfunction. Doctors recognized that they could use this as a therapeutic tool by controlling the amount of radiation exposure. Although exposure to high levels of radiation are linked to thyroid cancer, there has been no evidence since I^{131} treatment started that such a risk exists at radiation exposures at this level.

Your doctor will recommend that you use reliable birth control during I^{131} treatment. There are two reasons for this. One is that the radioactive iodine could affect the fetus. The other is that as the I^{131} begins to become effective, many people (men and women alike) find that any fertility problems associated with overactive thyroid disappear fairly immediately. If your fertility has been low for long enough that you haven't been using birth control, you could be in for a surprise! Even though the I^{131} is no longer in your body after five to seven days, it's still wise for women to delay efforts to become pregnant. This gives your body time to recover from the effects of overactive thyroid before it has to deal with the changes that accompany pregnancy.

Although you are somewhat radioactive for a week or so after you take the I^{131} capsule, it's not in any way noticeable to others or to you. Your doctor might recommend that you limit your exposure to young children and pregnant women for five days after you take your I^{131} dose, just as a precaution. Children and developing fetuses are very sensitive to many environmental exposures, which can have long-term effects when they alter the development process in some way. Drink lots of water during the first week of your treatment, to help flush the radioactive iodine out of your system.

You should notice that your thyroid gland (goiter) is smaller within three months of treatment. You should also start feeling better in regard to any symptoms of overactive thyroid. Doctors often prescribe beta blockers (discussed a little later in this chapter) to relieve some of these symptoms while you're waiting for the I^{131} to have an effect. Generally your doctor will then reduce or stop the beta blocker as you begin to feel better.

A single dose of radioactive iodine successfully ends hyperthyroidism for about 95 percent of people who use this treatment. If you are among the 5 percent for whom it doesn't, your doctor might repeat the I^{131} (in three to six months after the first dose), or might suggest a different treatment approach.

PROPYLTHIOURACIL (PTU)

Propylthiouracil, or PTU in medical shorthand, was the first of the antithyroid drugs to come into existence. It became available in the United States in the mid-1940s. It works by interfering with your thyroid gland's ability to make T4 and T3, and it only works while you are taking it. It takes two to ten weeks to notice an effect on your symptoms. The typical course of treatment is about two years. Although this is often enough to allow your natural thyroid balance to return to normal, about half the people who undergo this treatment find that their symptoms return within several months of ending the medication.

The most serious side effects of PTU are blood abnormalities, including decreased clotting time (which allows you to bleed longer before clots form). If you have heart disease or are taking an anticoagulant (blood thinner) it's generally unwise for you to take PTU, although you should discuss the complete advantages and disadvantages of this therapy with your doctor before making a decision. Do not take PTU if you are pregnant or breastfeeding.

PTU is administered at two dosing levels, initial and maintenance. The initial dose "loads" your system, establishing a baseline presence of the drug—a therapeutic level. Once your blood thyroid levels return to normal, a maintenance dose of PTU then keeps the drug's concentration in your blood at a therapeutic level.

These doses are not absolute! The dose that's right for you depends on your lab results and your symptoms. Take the dose your doctor prescribes, and take it according to the schedule your doctor tells you to follow. This drug is very sensitive, as is your body's response to it. Missing one dose usually is not a problem; just take the next one on schedule. If you miss two or more doses, let your doctor know.

Propylthiouracil (PTU) Dosing for Adults		
If your degree of hyperthyroidism is	The initial dose is usually	And the maintenance dose is usually
Mild	300 mg taken as a single dose or divided into three doses taken 8 hours apart	100 mg–150 mg daily
Moderate	600 mg taken as a single dose or divided into three doses taken 8 hours apart	150 mg–200 mg daily
Severe	900 mg taken as a single dose or divided into three doses taken 8 hours apart	200 mg–250 mg daily

METHIMAZOLE

Methimazole is sold under the brand name Tapazole. Like PTU, it prevents your thyroid gland from converting iodine and tyrosine into thyroid hormones (T3 and T4). However, methimazole also works to prevent T4 from converting to T3, which limits the amount of thyroid hormone that can enter your cells. Because of this dual action, methimazole begins to have an effect on hyperthyroid symptoms within days. Methimazole also is effective only during the time you are taking it, and has about the same rate of long-term effectiveness as PTU. Methimazole is about ten times more potent than PTU, although its actions are less consistent and its effects less predictable. Even with its rapid action, you need to take it for two years.

Methimazole does have some significant drawbacks. The most serious is a significant risk for permanent and potentially fatal liver damage. Another problem is its unpredictable degree of action. People absorb this drug inconsistently, which means the dose that is appropriate for one person might be too high or too low for someone else who has a similar degree of hyperthyroidism. Do not take methimazole if you are pregnant or breastfeeding.

The initial dose depends on how severe your hyperthyroidism is, and is given in three equal portions eight hours apart. You stay at this schedule until your thyroid hormone levels return to normal. Then your dose is adjusted to one-third to two-thirds of the initial dose, which you take daily for up to two years. Depending on your dose, your doctor might instruct you to split it into two doses taken twice daily. Pills come in strengths of 5 mg and 10 mg.

Methimazole Dosing for Adults		
If your degree of hyperthyroidism is	The initial dose is usually	And the maintenance dose is usually
Mild	5 mg taken three times daily (15 mg total each day)	5 mg–10 mg daily
Moderate	10 mg taken three times daily (30 mg total each day)	10 mg–20 mg daily
Severe	20 mg taken three times daily (60 mg total each day)	20 mg–40 mg daily

As with PTU, these doses are guidelines, not absolutes. Always take the dose your doctor prescribes, and take it according to the schedule your doctor tells you to follow. This drug is very sensitive, as is your body's response to it.

BETA BLOCKERS

The drugs known as beta blockers are so called because they block the "beta" receptors in your cells that ordinarily respond to the stimulating effect of epinephrine and norepinephrine. This response allows the physiological responses to take place that make you feel "wired" and nervous—increased heart rate and breathing rate, sweating, feeling of anxiety. Interfering with this response keeps these actions—and the symptoms they cause—from happening. Beta blockers have no direct effect on thyroid function.

Doctors often prescribe beta blockers in conjunction with drug therapy for hyperthyroidism because it takes so long for antithyroid drugs to have an effect. You usually stop taking the beta blocker once your blood thyroid levels return to normal and your symptoms go away. However, some beta blockers interact with PTU and methimazole. Such interactions can affect either or both drugs, so careful monitoring is important.

SURGERY TO SLOW THYROID FUNCTION

Surgery to remove the thyroid is called thyroidectomy. If just part of the thyroid is removed, which is the most common kind of surgery, it's called a partial thyroidectomy. If all of the thyroid gland is removed, it's called a total or complete thyroidectomy. For certain kinds of hyperthyroidism, surgery might be the treatment of first choice. These include:

- Tumors, particularly the rare tumors that are precancerous or cancerous
- Some toxic nodules

- Graves' disease that is producing severe symptoms at the time of diagnosis
- Graves' disease when you are under age 25, or when you want to become pregnant (in which case radiation therapy and drug therapy are too risky).
- Large goiters that interfere with swallowing or breathing

In other situations, surgery becomes an option when drug therapy (including radioactive iodine) fails. Nearly always, you must be euthyroid—at normal blood thyroid levels—before surgery. So doctors often prescribe drug therapy to suppress hyperthyroidism before doing surgery.

Thyroidectomy is done under general anesthesia. The surgeon makes an incision across the base of your neck, running the same direction as your collarbone and in a slight upward curve. This follows the natural lines and folds of your skin, so that after the incision fully heals, the scar is barely noticeable. Most people stay in the hospital for no longer than a few days, and can return to normal activities within two weeks. After partial thyroidectomy your blood thyroid levels might stay normal, although many people find that their levels decrease over time until hypothyroidism sets in. Hypothyroidism is certain after total thyroidectomy, and your doctor will start you on thyroid hormone replacement immediately after surgery. Except for hypothyroidism, and the usual risks of surgery, there are no long-term adverse effects from thyroidectomy.

TEMPORARY HYPERTHYROIDISM: REMOVING THE CAUSE

Sometimes environmental causes set up the situation of overactive thyroid. You can get too much iodine if you are taking thyroid hormone supplement to treat underactive thyroid and through dietary sources. Kelp and other kinds of seaweed, common in many dietary supplements, are high in iodine. Some people can handle extra dietary iodine without any untoward effects. In most people, their thyroid glands behave more like children gobbling candy—they continue to take in as much as is available, resulting in churning out far more thyroid hormone (T3 and T4) than the body needs.

As well, some dietary supplements promoted for weight loss, chronic tiredness, and "thyroid health" contain small amounts of desiccated thyroid extract as a "tonic." If you have an underactive thyroid, or the symptoms of underactive thyroid with normal lab results, you might be taking these supplements to boost your thyroid function. But it's easy to get too much of a good thing, particularly since government regulations for consistency of ingredients is far less stringent for nutritional products than for drugs. Such supplements are especially likely to cause problems if you are taking thyroid hormone supplement to treat underactive thyroid, leading to overdosing that results in overactive thyroid.

Some drugs interfere with thyroid function and create hyperthyroidism. The list of these is long, but includes certain drugs to treat conditions such as irregular heart rhythms and asthma, and even hormones such as birth control pills. For more about these kinds of interactions, see Chapter 13.

Fortunately it's easy for doctors to determine whether overactive thyroid is endogenous (caused by factors within your body) or environmental (caused by factors outside your body, such as foods or drugs). When the problem is endogenous, the radioactive iodine uptake test will show increased iodine uptake in your thyroid gland. When the problem is environmental, iodine uptake is normal or even low because your thyroid gland is "full." With rare exceptions, treatment is as simple as eliminating the environmental source.

NONPHARMACEUTICAL THERAPIES

Nearly all nonpharmaceutical therapies for thyroid imbalance target underactive rather than overactive thyroid. However, it is not uncommon for such therapies to end up causing hyperthyroidism. If you are taking nutritional supplements of any kind and you experience symptoms of overactive thyroid, stop taking the supplements and check the list of ingredients. Ask your doctor or pharmacist which of them might influence thyroid function. Some nutritional products, as we mentioned earlier, actually contain small amounts of desiccated thyroid extract as an "energizer." Unfortunately, this can energize you right into a serious health problem!

You can use some natural substances to help treat a hyperthyroid condition. High amounts of soy and soy-based protein can lower the conversion of T4 to T3. Also, certain bioflavonoids, particularly quercitin, can have a thyroid-lowering effect. One recent journal article suggests that the amino acid l-carnitine can be used to treat hyperthyroidism by slowing the conversion of T4 to T3. High doses of alpha-lipoic acid have also been used. However, a more comprehensive natural treatment for hyperthyroidism usually focuses on the autoimmune nature of this illness, by paying attention to the gut and its relationship to immunity, by withdrawing foods and other substances that may be adversely stimulating the immune system, by correcting nutrient imbalances, and by controlling symptoms by herbal and other measures. Only try this approach under medical supervision.

TRADITIONAL CHINESE MEDICINE (TCM) PERSPECTIVE

When your thyroid is overactive, this represents an imbalance in which yang dominates. Restoring the balance between yin and yang restores the balance of your thyroid's functions. Overactive thyroid represents a deficiency of yin and an excess of yang. The traditional Chinese medicine practitioner might make one of three diagnoses for someone with hyperthyroidism:

- Kidney Yin Deficiency with Excess Heat—In addition to enlarged thyroid gland, typical symptoms include anger, anxiety, flushed face, dry mouth, tremor, rapid pulse, increased appetite, and heat intolerance.
- Yin Deficiency with Heart and Liver Deficiency—In addition to enlarged thyroid gland, typical symptoms include dry throat, heart palpitations, trouble sleeping, weight loss, and rapid but weak pulse.
- Yin Deficiency with Heart and Kidney Deficiency—In addition to enlarged thyroid gland, typical symptoms include dry eyes, fertility difficulties (men and women), dry mouth, rapid pulse, and heart palpitations. TCM remedies vary with the precise diagnosis, and typically include the herbs rehmannia (shu di huang), dioscorea (shan yao), and cornus (shan zhu yu). Some TCM practitioners might use kidney yin tonic (liu wei di huang wan), liver cleansing (zhi zi qing gan tang), and heart yin tonic (tian wang bu xin dan) formulas, depending on the TCM diagnosis.

Acupuncture can be useful in controlling the symptoms of hyperthyroidism, particularly the racing heart, anxiety, and heat intolerance. Needles usually are placed with a "dispersion" technique, meaning that the needles are retained and the patient lies still, allowing energy to disperse or calm down. There are several different acupuncture systems being used currently in the United States, but many of them would include treatment of the heart and Triple Warmer channels. Called "Fire" energy for their heat and activity-stimulating effects, disharmony in these channels can lead to many of the symptoms associated with hyperthyroidism. Also common is strengthening of the Kidney or Water channel, because water will help to cool down fire. Some acupuncture techniques include so-called microsystems such as ear acupuncture, that can assist in symptom control.

WHEN SOMETHING ELSE IS THE CAUSE OF YOUR SYMPTOMS

Most of the time, thyroid function tests provide conclusive evidence of hyperthyroidism. Unlike hypothyroidism, when this evidence is lacking but you have the symptoms of overactive thyroid the cause is usually something other than thyroid imbalance. You might have an imbalance elsewhere in your endocrine matrix, or might be getting too many stimulants in your diet. Caffeine and decongestant medications are common stimulant culprits. It's important to evaluate your symptoms and your blood-test results to make an accurate diagnosis before you begin treatment.

12

Therapeutic Balance: Finding the Right Treatment for You

Doctors want to help people. That's why they're doctors. Nothing makes a doctor happier than having you come back for a follow-up visit to report that your symptoms are gone and you feel great. And about 60 percent of the time, this is the result with thyroid imbalance. Your doctor makes a diagnosis, gives you a prescription, and within a few months you're back to your usual energetic, vibrant self. Now if this were baseball, this would be an outstanding batting average! But it's not baseball. It's not a game at all. It's your health, your life. You want—and deserve—better results. Nearly everyone can get better results. For some of you, however, it's going to take time to find the right therapeutic balance.

MULTIPLE AND CHANGING TREATMENT OPTIONS

Once upon a time, there was just one treatment for thyroid dysfunction: dried and ground thyroid gland extracted from sheep, pigs, and cows. The only problem was, you never really knew how much you were getting. One batch might leave you almost manic, while another batch left you unable to avoid an afternoon nap every day. Then along came Synthroid, pure and clean and made entirely in a laboratory. And most important, consistent (mostly). The availability of eleven dosage strengths helped your doctor tailor a prescription to fit your needs. Doctors and patients were happy (mostly), and Synthroid became the standard of treatment for underactive thyroid.

That was 40 years ago! Yet levothyroxine (Synthroid and similar thyroid hormone supplement products) remains the standard of treatment that many doctors still follow. If it is a treatment that works for you, that's great. It does work just fine for many people with underactive thyroid. But it's no longer the only trick in the bag, so to speak. There are many treatment options available today. They include:

- Levothyroxine alone (Synthroid and similar products)
- Levothyroxine along with T3 (Cytomel)
- Natural desiccated thyroid (Armour and similar products) alone
- Natural desiccated thyroid along with T3
- T3 alone, either Cytomel or compounded slow-release forms
- Any of the above, along with support for adrenal function

As well, there are numerous ways to support your thyroid's function and health through diet, activity, herbs, and nutritional supplements (see Chapter 15). Today, treatment for thyroid is a matter of choices, not just following a standard that could be older than you are.

BALANCE IS DYNAMIC

We're recognizing, too, that therapeutic balance is dynamic. As your life changes—you gain or lose weight, change your eating habits, change your activity level, develop other health conditions, or just plain grow older—the changes affect your entire metabolic matrix, and with it your thyroid function. Keeping your thyroid, and the rest of your endocrine system, in balance requires shifting your treatment to accommodate the changes in your life. In an ideal world, you would see your doctor once a year for a full assessment of your thyroid status, including a complete thyroid panel, thorough physical examination, and other lab tests that might be relevant (such as adrenal function or estrogen and FSH levels if you're at menopause age). What happens in the real world seldom comes close!

Once your thyroid balance becomes stable, usually you and your doctor forget about it. Out of sight, out of mind. Everything's working fine, it seems, so why look for problems? What usually happens goes like this: your doctor comes in, feels your neck, asks how you're doing, listens long enough to hear you say, "fine," gives you a lab slip for a T4 and perhaps a TSH, authorizes prescription refills for another year, and you're out the door.

But what if you're not fine, really? Do you know this? Sometimes not. Doctors often ask broad questions, believing this encourages you to respond openly and freely, without feeling squeezed into a particular kind of answer. "How are you feeling?" gives you wide latitude, while "Does it hurt when you swallow?" requires a specific, limited response. But sometimes it's those specific, limited responses that provide clues that things are not quite fine. You might not think about how your throat feels when you swallow, especially if you have a low-level discomfort you've had for long enough that you've learned to ignore it. Having your doctor specifically ask, though, brings it to your awareness again.

If you answer "yes" to the question about whether it hurts when you swallow, this gives your doctor a line of questioning and examination to pursue. Maybe you breathe through your mouth, which dries your throat tissues. Maybe you have chronic tonsillitis. Maybe your thyroid gland is a bit swollen or has a nodule, and pushes back against your esophagus when you swallow. In any case, your response gives your doctor paths to follow to evaluate your thyroid function as well as other potential health concerns.

Other specific questions give thyroid-specific information, too. "How's your energy level?" is nicely general, and might get you to say that you feel fine after your third cup of coffee in the morning, or to comment that life with three kids, a demanding boss, and a 45-minute commute doesn't leave much energy for anything. Or you might just say, "Fine, mostly."

Although responses along the lines of the first two should arouse your doctor's interest and lead to further questioning, they might instead lead to shared commiseration! But "Do you still feel tired when you wake up in the morning?" is certain to get a specific response from you, and your answer is a clue to one of the key signs of adrenal stress, which might suggest underactive thyroid or at the very least an endocrine imbalance.

BECOME YOUR OWN ADVOCATE

It might seem obvious, but you must be your own advocate when it comes to matters of your thyroid and your health. Practically speaking, it's just not possible for your doctor to keep up with *every* development in medicine. So doctors choose to keep up with the developments that affect the greatest percentages of their patients. If your doctor treats a lot of people with thyroid imbalance, then he or she probably keeps up with research results, gene therapy concepts, and other new treatment approaches. If not . . .

Keep a record of how you feel—write notes or write in a journal. This gives you a perspective over time of how well your treatment regimen is working for you. Perhaps you schedule your annual doctor's appointment during vacation time, so you don't have to take off from work or school. But you're also likely to be better rested and more relaxed because you're away from the daily details of your life. When your doctor says, "So how are you doing?" you can say "Fine!" and mean it. Two weeks ago, however, you might've found it difficult to make it through the afternoons.

Keeping a record also helps you monitor circumstances and situations that make your thyroid balance better or worse, giving you insights into the kinds of lifestyle changes you might make to better support your thyroid and your endocrine matrix. The more we learn about thyroid function and balance, the more we recognize how integrated and interrelated everything is. Therapeutic balance is really life balance.

ASSESSING YOUR THYROID STATUS

Before your next regular appointment with your doctor to assess your thyroid status, do a little assessing of your own. This will help you be prepared for your visit and ready to share any concerns that you have. If you haven't been keeping a thyroid or health journal, it's not too late to start. Don't make this into a chore (we all know what happens when good intentions become chores!), but try to establish some consistency. Write a few notes at least once a week about how you feel and what things are happening in your life. For example, do periods of short-term stress, such as final exams at school or a big deadline at work, affect how you feel? Write specific details and examples.

Here are some other factors to assess before your next doctor's visit:

- How long have you been taking thyroid hormone supplement? If five years or longer, consider talking with your doctor about treatment options now available and whether there is any reason for you to make a change.

- Have you been taking the same brand since you started treatment? If you're satisfied with the brand of thyroid hormone supplement that you take, there's not necessarily any reason to change. Some people are shocked to find out, however, that there are several levothyroxine products available and that they are significantly cheaper than Synthroid. You can change brands, as long as your doctor runs a follow-up blood test to make sure your blood thyroid levels are where they should be. The best approach is to do blood tests before making the change and then two to six weeks after making the change, so you can make an accurate comparison.

- Have you been taking the same dose since you started treatment? Your thyroid hormone needs change over time, as does whatever thyroid function you still have. If your dose has been the same for five years or longer, ask your doctor to run a complete thyroid panel instead of just T4/TSH, so you can get a comprehensive picture of your thyroid function. This will give you and your doctor more information for assessing whether your dose is appropriate.

- Is your daily dose of levothyroxine 125 mcg or higher? We now know that most people don't need doses higher than this (although some do, so don't worry if you're one of them) to maintain adequate blood thyroid levels. Higher doses of thyroid hormone supplement raise your risk for calcium loss and osteoporosis, so if you need a higher dose, talk with your doctor about ways to offset this potential problem.

- Do you adjust your thyroid hormone supplement dose on your own? Some people make changes in how much levothyroxine they take based on how they feel. This is not a good idea! If you take more than your prescribed dose because it gives you an energy boost during times of stress, then your dose might be too low. If you take your levothyroxine just five days a week instead of seven because you feel jittery by the fifth day, then your dose is probably too high. You might do better with a combination of T4 and T3 supplement, with T3 to meet short-term thyroid hormone needs and T4 for long-term stability.

- What changes have taken place in your life or lifestyle since you were first diagnosed with hypothyroidism? Eating habits, activity levels, stress levels, pregnancy, menopause, and health problems all affect thyroid function.

- Does your doctor order just T4 and TSH blood tests, or a complete thyroid panel? For years the standard follow-up has been T4/TSH monitoring, with additional tests if the results were borderline or questionable. But T4/TSH levels alone don't present a very complete picture.

- Have you begun to take estrogen replacement therapy, or other medications that interfere with thyroid absorption and function? Thyroid function should always be retested after initiating such therapy.

Most doctors appreciate a collaborative approach to health care, and are willing to discuss different treatment approaches or at least explain their reasons for the approaches they prefer. Doctors, like everyone else, are creatures of habit. Yours might consistently prescribe Synthroid because that's just what he or she has always done. Perhaps your doctor tried T3 therapy with a patient and had a bad outcome, and now is leery of using it again. There are many reasons that doctors choose treatment approaches, and not all of them necessarily have anything to do with your specific circumstances.

CHANGING THE STANDARD

As doctors are learning more about how the thyroid functions and how thyroid hormone affects other body functions, they're becoming more receptive to, and even interested in, exploring new treatment approaches. Many of what we could call mainstream doctors are reluctant to try T3 supplementation or natural desiccated thyroid. They view these as alternative approaches. And indeed, the doctors who are more likely to suggest these therapies are more inclined toward complementary or holistic medicine. But the mainstream is slowly shifting as doctors recognize that the problems they associate with these treatments are no longer valid reasons to avoid trying them.

PHYSICIAN RESISTANCE TO PRESCRIBING NATURAL DESICCATED THYROID

Forty years ago the hormone content of desiccated thyroid extract was highly variable and produced unpredictable results. And yes, from batch to batch desiccated thyroid extract is still less consistent than are synthetic products. But these differences are generally within what we consider to be clinically tolerable. That is to say, they don't matter for the vast majority of people who take these products. If your thyroid levels are extraordinarily volatile, you might be among those for whom this inconsistency is a problem. But if your thyroid levels are *that* volatile, odds are high that there are other health problems at work.

A recent point of concern about natural desiccated thyroid extract has been its source. In the old days, thyroid extract came from various animal thyroid glands, most commonly from cows. When "mad cow disease" struck in the 1990s, any product related to cows became suspect. Thyroid extract was among these products, and for good reason: glandular tissues, scientists believe, are at high risk for carrying the infectious agent responsible for this devastating disease.

"Mad cow disease," known officially as bovine spongiform encephalopathy (BSE), is a brain-wasting infection that affects only cows. But the infection can cause a related disease in humans, called variant Creutzfeldt-Jakob disease (vCJD). Although vCJD is very rare, it is always fatal. People get vCJD by consuming products from cows infected with BSE. There is no way to test for the presence of BSE in bovine products. Armour, Westhroid, and Nature-Throid brands of natural desiccated thyroid are porcine, or from pig sources. This eliminates any risk associated with BSE. All USP thyroid products should be of porcine origin, but sticking to brand-name products is one way of assuring this. If you have any doubts, ask the pharmacist to confirm the product's origin.

Products sold as nutritional supplements could contain bovine thyroid extract. Read labels carefully. If the label says the source is bovine or if the label doesn't list the source, don't buy the product. Although the risk is minimal, preventing it is as simple as not using the product.

PHYSICIAN RESISTANCE TO PRESCRIBING T3 SUPPLEMENT

T3 is significantly more potent than T4, the ingredient in levothyroxine, and rapid-acting. Because of this, doctors tend to consider T3 supplement a less reliable method for managing hypothyroidism. You need to take T3 twice a day (or even three times a day, depending on the dose). It goes straight to the cell, so it has an effect almost immediately. This causes doctors to worry about overdosing.

T3 supplementation isn't for everyone. If you're stable and feel fine on T4 (natural desiccated or levothyroxine), there's no reason to add T3 (sold as the brand-name product Cytomel in the United States) to your treatment regimen. T3 supplementation is most effective for people who have trouble finding balance with

T4 supplementation, and also who are willing to take T3 on a fairly rigid schedule. But for the majority of people who use T3, overdosing is a very slight risk. Symptoms of a dose that's too high include jitters, heart palpitations, sweating, and sometimes nausea. They generally pass within six to eight hours. If you experience such symptoms, call your doctor before your next T3 dose.

Your doctor might prescribe low-dose T3 supplementation alone if your thyroid blood hormone levels seem normal but you have symptoms of underactive thyroid. If you have clinical hypothyroidism—your blood thyroid hormone levels are abnormal—T3 alone is usually not adequate to give you consistent thyroid hormone levels. When you choose to try T3 supplementation, whether alone or in combination with T4, be prepared to spend some time trying to find the right dose. You might also find that the dose you need can vary according to other factors in your life, such as stress or dietary changes. Some doctors have begun to prescribe low-dose T3 for specific health problems such as hair loss and mild depression. Research is beginning to support this use, even in the face of normal thyroid test results.

FINDING THE THERAPEUTIC BALANCE THAT'S RIGHT FOR YOU

Remember that balance is dynamic. It changes. What works for you now might not be so effective in five years. What didn't work for you five years ago might be just the ticket now. Finding therapeutic balance with thyroid treatment is an ongoing process of vigilance and adjustment. For most people, there is no one approach that will carry you from diagnosis through the rest of your life.

It's important for you to stay up on the latest research findings and thinking as far as thyroid treatment goes. It's just as important to find a doctor who does the same—and who is willing to collaborate with you to find treatment approaches that are consistent not only with your clinical picture but also your personal philosophy about health (and taking care of it) and your lifestyle. It's also important to make decisions about your thyroid balance and your health based on your symptoms and circumstances, rather than leaping to try the treatment du jour just because it's new. Certainly, many people with thyroid imbalance are stuck on old treatment regimens and would do much better with an updated approach. But don't feel compelled to make changes just for the sake of change. Make sure there is at least one sound therapeutic advantage to the new approach. Right now, there is no cure for underactive thyroid. But there is management, and effective management can give you the balance you seek—for your thyroid function, for your endocrine matrix, for your health in general, and for your life. Even when your thyroid function is normal by standard measurements, there are lifestyle modifications that can help to improve the metabolic effects of the body's thyroid. Eating enough protein will ensure that l-tyrosine will be available to make thyroglobulin, and iodine intake is an issue for some. Other nutrients such as zinc, selenium, and vitamin A are involved in the conversion of T4 to its active form, T3. Exercise and stress reduction seem to have positive effects. And attention to allergens in the diet can lower immune system activation, lessening the possibility of autoantibodies to thyroid and other tissues.

13

What Do You Do When Nothing Seems to Work?

No treatment approach is without the risk of problems or failure, and thyroid therapy is no exception. One of the most frustrating dimensions of thyroid imbalance is the difficulty in finding a treatment regimen that fully relieves your symptoms. This is primarily a factor when the problem is underactive thyroid, which is often insidious and long-term in its onset. By the time you get a diagnosis (if, in fact, you even do), your body has tried everything it knows to adapt to the low levels of thyroid hormone. This, of course, throws other body functions out of balance as well, altering your body's homeostasis, or state of equilibrium.

As treatment begins to restore balance to your thyroid, these other functions are still "set" at compensatory levels. They have been "normal" within the framework of dysfunction that has evolved within your body. Now that treatment is shifting your thyroid balance, these other functions are again out of sync. They, too, must realign. This isn't always easy, and sometimes needs a boost in terms of implementing temporary treatment such as for adrenal fatigue, as we discussed in Chapter 8. Finding balance becomes an extended process of adjustment among the various components of your endocrine matrix.

LOOKING FOR ANSWERS

Finding a balanced approach to thyroid dysfunction can be an extended process. Sometimes it's an accumulation of the little things that add up to disappointment. The questions in the following sections can help you identify the "stones in the path" that could be keeping your chosen approach from achieving the thyroid balance you desire. Answer all of the questions completely and honestly, so that you get a true assessment of your thyroid situation.

ASSESSMENT SECTION 1: THE CURRENT STATE OF YOUR THYROID

The first step in determining why your current thyroid treatment regimen might not be working for you, or in finding out if you can fine-tune your regimen for even better results, is to assess your current thyroid status. Many people complain that they still have symptoms, but either have been on thyroid treatment for less than six months or have not had a full follow-up medical assessment for several years. Just running TSH and T4 levels once a year before your doctor renews your prescription doesn't really count as assessment.

1. *What is your thyroid diagnosis (original and secondary, if this applies to you)?*
2. *When did you receive your thyroid diagnosis?* How long you've had thyroid imbalance can influence how well conventional treatments work for you. Sometimes people develop thyroid resistance, in which the thyroid gland becomes less responsive to thyroid hormone supplement. As well, thyroid hormone needs change as you get older. There's more on these topics later in this chapter.
3. *What are your most recent blood thyroid levels?*

4. *On what date were they drawn?*

5. *What time of the day were they drawn?* Once stabilized on a treatment regimen, many people receive only basic follow-up lab tests to determine whether thyroid hormone levels in the blood are within normal ranges. Thyroid test results are most "true" when your blood is drawn right before your supplement dose is due and before you've had anything to eat or drink. Lab technicians are supposed to note the time of the blood draw and ask you when you last ate, but this information doesn't always make it to your doctor at the same time your blood results do. Your doctor often receives test results electronically, with the full paper record following several days to several weeks later.

6. *What symptoms are you having and how long have you had them?*

7. *How have your symptoms changed over the last six months?*

8. *How have your symptoms changed over the last 12 months?*

9. *How have your symptoms changed since you were first diagnosed with thyroid imbalance?* Very little in your life stays the same for very long, and your thyroid balance is no exception. If you take thyroid hormone supplement or have symptoms of thyroid imbalance, keep a thyroid journal. At least once a month, write down how you're feeling and what symptoms, if any, that you've been having. If you do start to have problems, this gives you a running record to show to your doctor.

10. *Which option best describes your doctor's approach to thyroid problems?*

☐ "Here's a prescription. I want you to take one pill every morning and call me in six months."

Disinterested, feels that thyroid imbalance is more of a nuisance than a "real" medical problem. Hasn't listened to anything you've said.

☐ "Let's run a couple of blood tests and see where things are. If your thyroid levels are off, we'll start you on some medication."
Follows convention, looks for tangible evidence.

☐ "Tell me how you feel as you go through the day."
Interested in hearing your unique experience.

☐ "There's been a lot of research about thyroid function lately, and we have new information and treatment approaches. Let's start with a complete set of lab tests, and then talk about your symptoms. Here's a health and lifestyle questionnaire to get you started."
Stays up on the latest developments, follows current research, remains open to doing things differently and to breaking from convention when it's in the patient's (your) best interests.

11. *What thyroid hormone supplement(s) are you currently taking?*

12. *How long have you been taking this drug (these drugs)?*
The longer you've been on treatment for thyroid imbalance, the more comfortable you and your doctor become about your treatment regimen. This is especially true when you've been seeing the same doctor since your diagnosis. Doctors, like the rest of us, tend to leave well enough alone. If you seem to be doing okay or have what your doctor thinks are minor or "to be expected" symptoms and complaints, you're probably still on the same thyroid hormone supplement product and dose that you were taking when your blood levels stabilized after starting treatment.

13. *What time of day do you take your thyroid supplement?*
14. *Do you take it before you eat, after you eat, or with some kind of food (including coffee or tea)?* How and when you take your thyroid hormone supplement is as important as what you take. If you are taking levothyroxine (such as Synthroid, Levothroid, Unithroid) or desiccated thyroid (such as Armour), results are most consistent when you take it at the same time every day and at least two hours before or after any food or beverages (except water). Doctors usually prescribe T3 in equal doses to be taken two or three times a day. This regimen is most effective when you take your doses by the clock: every 8 hours for three-times-a-day dosing, and every 12 hours for twice-daily dosing.

ASSESSMENT SECTION 2: OTHER HEALTH PROBLEMS

Other health problems can affect your thyroid balance, and your thyroid balance can affect other health problems. Short-term, episodic conditions such as viral infections also can have short-term effects on your thyroid balance. Frequent viral infections suggest that your immune system might not be working as effectively as it could. Health problems that affect your endocrine matrix are especially likely to interact with thyroid function.

1. *What other health conditions do you have?* This is a small question with big ramifications. Other autoimmune and endocrine disorders are often intimately interrelated with thyroid function and dysfunction. Treating one changes the balance of all. It's important to coordinate and integrate treatment across the endocrine matrix instead of focusing on individual symptom sets.
2. *What is your BMI?* (See page 227 if you don't know, or just write down your height and weight.) Being over-

weight affects the way your body absorbs and uses many drugs. It also affects your general health, and is a key contributing factor to numerous health problems often connected with thyroid imbalance, such as diabetes.

3. *How much weight have you lost and/or gained over the past 12 months?* Count each episode of gain and each episode of loss. Cycles of weight loss and gain confuse your body's systems. They might also signal fluctuating thyroid hormone levels; when your weight is up your thyroid is down, and when your weight is down your thyroid is up. This could result from many variables, including changes in your eating and activity habits, variations in your thyroid hormone supplement from prescription to prescription, or the influence of other endocrine imbalances such as adrenal fatigue or type 2 diabetes. Weight changes of greater than 10 percent (either gain or loss) also can affect the amount of thyroid hormone supplement that you need to take.

ASSESSMENT SECTION 3: OTHER PRESCRIPTION DRUGS

Prescription drugs that you take for other health conditions can interact with thyroid hormone supplement. The drugs can affect each other's absorption and effectiveness, either reducing or intensifying the intended results. Oral medications for diabetes reduce the effectiveness of thyroid hormone supplement. So do products containing estrogen, such as birth control pills (oral contraceptives) and hormone replacement therapy (HRT). Cholesterol-lowering drugs bind with the thyroid hormone in thyroid supplements, preventing the thyroid hormone from entering your bloodstream. And if you're taking a tricyclic antidepressant and thyroid hormone supplement, each drug is likely to increase the effects of the other.

1. *What other prescription drugs do you take?*
2. *When do you take these other drugs?*
3. *Do you take more than one drug at the same time? If so, what combinations?* How and when you take drugs is as significant as what you take. When you pick up a prescription from the pharmacy, tell the pharmacist what other drugs you're taking and ask if there are any interactions you should watch for or changes you should make in the ways you take them. Do the same thing with your doctor whenever he or she prescribes a new medication. Many other prescription drugs interfere with the absorption of thyroid hormone supplement from your intestines into your bloodstream or with its action once in your system. They include:

Amiodarone (slows heart rate)
Androgens and anabolic hormones
Asparaginase
Carbamazepine
Chloral hydrate
Cholestyramine
Clofibrate
Diazepam
Dopamine and dopamine agonists (drugs to treat heart problems and Parkinson's disease)
Estrogen (in birth control pills or hormone replacement therapy)
Ethionamide
Furosemide (diuretic)
Glucocorticoids
Heparin
Insulin
Levodopa
Lithium (bipolar disorder)
Lovastatin
Meclofenamic acid
Mefenamic acid
Methadone
Metoclopramide
Mitotane
Nitroprusside
Nonsteroidal anti-inflammatory agents (arthritis, inflammation)
Perphenazine
Phenobarbital
Phenylbutazone
Phenytoin (antiseizure)
Resorcinol
Rifampin
Somatostatin analogs
Sulfonamides
Sulfonylureas (oral medication for diabetes such as glipizide, glucotrol, glyburide)
Tamoxifen
Thiazide diuretics (such as hydrochlorodiazide)

ASSESSMENT SECTION 4: OVER-THE-COUNTER PRODUCTS, HERBAL REMEDIES, AND NUTRITIONAL SUPPLEMENTS

Over-the-counter drugs such as pain relievers, allergy preparations, and even antacids also can interact with thyroid hormone supplement. And though you might not think of herbal remedies and nutritional supplements as drugs, they do contain chemical substances that alter body functions. In particular, products that contain kelp, a common filler, are high in iodine, which suppresses thyroid function.

1. *What over-the-counter drugs, supplements, and remedies (such as pain relievers, allergy products, and laxatives) do you use on a regular basis (i.e., three times a week or more)?* Salicylates (such as aspirin and Pepto-Bismol), calcium, nonsteroidal anti-inflammatory drugs, aluminum hydroxide (antacid), and ferrous sulfate (iron supplement) are among the over-the-counter substances that can interact with thyroid hormone supplement. These substances are in a wide variety of products including pain relievers, laxatives, vitamins, cold and flu preparations, and remedies for upset stomach. The aluminum in liquid antacids binds with the thyroid hormone, rendering it fairly ineffective. Noninflammatory steroids (NSAIDs) and aspirin also reduce the effectiveness of thyroid supplement.

2. *For what reasons do you use these products?* Not only can the products interact with thyroid hormone or affect thyroid function, but taking them regularly can mask symptoms that you should check out. Persistent headaches, gastrointestinal upset, and other problems could signal underlying health issues.

3. *What herbal supplements do you take that are marketed specifically for thyroid health?*

4. *What herbal supplements do you take that are marketed for increased energy, improved sex drive, or improved memory and alertness?* These products often contain small amounts of desiccated thyroid extract, which add to the effect of your thyroid supplement. Kelp and seaweed, substances high in iodine, are common fillers in many herbal and nutritional supplement products. Taking them regularly can suppress thyroid function, making it seem that your thyroid hormone supplement dose is too low.

5. *Do you drink herbal tea or green tea?* Green tea has numerous health benefits. It also has a moderate to high amount of caffeine, depending on how long it's brewed before serving. Caffeine is a stimulant that has many effects on the body's metabolic functions. Herbal teas can contain unexpected ingredients that can interfere with how your body absorbs and uses thyroid hormone replacement; always read the labels.

ASSESSMENT SECTION 5: EATING HABITS

The foods you eat become the fuel for your body's functions. Food in general, and certain foods in particular, can interfere with how well your system absorbs thyroid hormone supplement. (See Chapter 15 for a discussion of foods that have a direct effect on thyroid function and thyroid hormone levels in your body.)

1. *When is the first time in the day that you typically have something to eat or drink?*

2. *What is the first item of food or drink that you consume in a typical day?* If you take your supplement when you get up in the morning, is it two hours before you eat? For best absorption, it should be, but you might not give

yourself that much preparation time in the morning. Many breakfast foods are fortified with calcium, which interferes with absorption. And that morning caffeine jolt affects your metabolism in many ways—which is, of course, one reason you start your day with coffee or tea, but also could create problems with your thyroid balance. Caffeine is a diuretic, which means that it pulls fluid from your body. This alters your chemical balances, and puts a particular stress on your adrenal glands.

3. *What is the last time in the day that you typically have something to eat or drink?* Eating within four hours of going to bed is likely to interfere with your sleep patterns, since all that food is stocking your body's energy stores. This can affect the rhythms of your endocrine matrix, from cortisol to melatonin and the other hormones involved in circadian rhythms. Altering these hormonal functions correspondingly alters thyroid functions, from thyroid hormone production in the thyroid gland to T4-to-T3 conversion in the liver and cells.

4. *Do you eat regular meals spaced evenly throughout the day?*

5. *What do you typically eat and drink for snacks during the day?*

6. *What have you had to eat today? (List everything, including snacks and beverages.)* Eating regularly throughout the day maintains a consistent flow of nutrients to your body, minimizing metabolic fluctuations. If you eat little during the day, you're likely to be famished by evening—and likely to eat more food overall than if you'd eaten regularly through the day. This is a pattern that's disruptive to your body rhythms, and also that contributes to weight control challenges.

7. *How many servings a day do you eat of fruits, veg-etables, and whole grain products? Do you eat the same amount of servings every day?* These foods are high in fiber, and fiber affects both the rate at which foods travel through your digestive system and the way nutrients and drugs are absorbed into your bloodstream. A diet relatively high in fiber is gener-ally good for your overall health. Its benefits are highest when the amount of fiber is consistent from day to day. This is also optimal if you take thyroid hormone supplement, because it helps to assure reli-able absorption.

8. *How much water do you drink each day?* An adult should drink between 8 and 12 glasses of water (8 ounces each) each day. Water is more essential to your body than food. Keeping yourself well hydrated helps all body systems to function at their best. It also helps you to get consistent absorption of thyroid hormone supplement.

9. *How many foods containing sugar, refined carbohy-drates, and white flour do you eat each day?* These foods stimulate insulin in the body, leading to a condi-tion called insulin resistance. The resulting insulin ele-vation can lead to diabetes type 2, early heart disease, weight increases, and depression. Metabolic abnormali-ties, including thyroid problems, can also result from reliance on these foods.

ASSESSMENT SECTION 6: ACTIVITY HABITS

Regular physical activity keeps your cells functioning at peak efficiency. But most of us don't get enough of it. Adults should get a minimum of 30 minutes of moderate physical activity, such as walking, at least four days a week. For optimal health, add 30 to 60 minutes of moderate to strenuous exercise each week.

1. *How far do you walk to work or school, or from where you park your car to your office or classroom?* Walking is one of the most effective ways to gently exercise your whole body, and it's easy to incorporate into your daily routine. If you take public transportation, get off at the stop before yours and walk the rest of the way. If you drive, park at the back of the lot and walk the extra distance. Look for other opportunities to walk throughout the day. Take the stairs instead of the elevator, and walk instead of drive to lunch.

2. *What level of activity does it take to get you to the point of feeling winded?* A healthy adult with no serious health problems should be able to walk up three flights of stairs without becoming winded.

3. *What is the most strenuous physical activity that you do in a typical week, and how often do you do it?*

4. *What physical activity do you most enjoy? How often do you get to do it?*

5. *What keeps you from being as active as you'd like to be?* You're most likely to participate in regular physical activity when you like what you're doing. Although on the surface this seems like common sense, a surprising number of people force themselves to do activities that they don't like. If you don't like jogging, then try brisk walking, in-line skating, bicycling, or swimming. These are all of comparable intensity, and will give you an equally effective workout.

ASSESSMENT SECTION 7: OTHER LIFESTYLE FACTORS

1. *Do you smoke?* Cigarette smoke contains many chemicals that cause a range of health problems, from minor to life-threatening. These chemicals affect body function at the cell level, causing changes that alter metabolism. Some research suggests that some of the chemicals in cigarette smoke directly damage thyroid cells. If you smoke, it will become increasingly difficult to maintain a thyroid balance.

2. *How much alcohol do you drink?* Drinking more than two drinks a day can damage liver function. This affects other body functions, and also directly affects peripheral T4-to-T3 conversion, which takes place in the liver.

3. *What caffeinated beverages, and how many of them, do you drink each day (coffee, tea, cola)?* Caffeine is a stimulant, which affects your metabolism. If your thyroid hormone supplement dose is a little too high, caffeine stimulation can send your symptoms over the edge.

4. *What time do you usually go to bed at night?*

5. *What time do you usually get up in the morning?* The typical adult needs 7 to 9 hours of sleep a night, yet studies show that the average amount of sleep most people get each night is closer to 5½ or 6 hours. Inadequate sleep triggers the hormones related to stress, which in turn influences thyroid hormone.

6. *Do you feel rested when you wake up?*

7. *Do you sleep in on weekends or days that you don't have to work or go to school?* Problems sleeping and feeling tired even after what should be adequate amounts asleep suggests underactive thyroid. If you're already taking thyroid hormone supplement, your dose might need to be increased.

SOMETIMES IT'S THE DRUG, NOT YOU

The fluctuations of the human body present challenge enough for maintaining thyroid balance. But the very substances you take to restore your body's balance might themselves be inconsistent. Hormones are not the most stable of chemical substances to begin with. Even synthetic hormones—those created in the laboratory—cannot be manufactured with precise accuracy. Natural hormone sources—desiccated thyroid from animal sources—are even less consistent from batch to batch.

There is potency variation among brands, too. Even though all of the levothyroxine products contain the same amount of levothyroxine for the same strength, each product uses different fillers and compounding processes that affect how the pill dissolves in your gastrointestinal tract. This is why doctors and pharmacists recommend staying with the same brand once you start taking a thyroid hormone supplement and find that it seems to work for you. It's also the reason you might have a reaction to one brand but not to another.

Although these sound like serious problems, for most people who take thyroid hormone supplement the inconsistencies aren't noticeable. Your body itself isn't consistent, either. Its needs for thyroid hormone change literally from minute to minute. But over 24 hours, a week, or a month, those needs average out. Targeting the average achieves balance.

If you are among the people whose thyroid balance is fragile, however, targeting the average isn't quite good enough. Those manufacturing variations do make a difference for you. The synthetic supplements such as levothyroxine (Synthroid and other brands) are more stable than the natural hormone products (Armour and other brands) despite the recent furor about their composition and consistency. You'll need to work with your doctor to find the right product or combination of products to achieve your personal thyroid balance. You also should explore imbalances other than thyroid, such as those that result from adrenal fatigue.

THYROID RESISTANCE

Sometimes your thyroid itself resists balance. Perhaps it has functioned in imbalance for so long that it can no longer redefine its own state of homeostasis. Generally when thyroid resistance exists, you have slightly unusual lab results. The changes can be subtle and perplexing. There appears to be a genetic involvement with most thyroid resistance that affects the hypothalamus-pituitary-thyroid matrix.

It's important to rule out interactions with other drugs before concluding the problem is thyroid resistance and adjusting your thyroid supplement regimen. The symptoms of thyroid resistance can mimic the symptoms of pituitary tumors, so your doctor will probably run tests to determine whether this is the underlying problem (very rare). Treatment might involve drugs to alter pituitary function, in addition to thyroid hormone supplement.

THYROID BALANCE AS YOU AGE

Thyroid function shifts with increasing age, too. Health experts now recommend baseline thyroid testing at age 35, to be repeated every three to five years until age 50. After age 50, you should have your blood thyroid levels checked once a year. The numbers tell the story:

- Ten percent of women age 50 and older have clinical hypothyroidism.
- Seventeen percent of women and 8 percent of men age 60 and older have clinical hypothyroidism.
- Three percent of men age 60 have clinical hyperthyroidism.

Other health changes take place with aging, too, that can confuse or even mask thyroid imbalance. Some of the symptoms of menopause—mood swings, irritability, tiredness, insomnia—are the same symptoms that suggest thyroid imbalance. Some health experts believe that most of what we identify as mild to moderate age-related dementia—the memory lapses and confusion we correlate with "old" age—are actually symptoms of thyroid imbalance. The rate of conditions such as depression is much higher in people over age 65 than under; coupled with the increased risk of thyroid imbalance, it's likely that thyroid function accounts for a good percentage of these.

The best thing you can do for your thyroid health after age 50 is to follow the recommendation to have your blood thyroid levels checked every year. If you have any symptoms of either overactive or underactive thyroid, have your doctor evaluate your thyroid status. If your lab results come back within normal ranges but you still have symptoms, ask your doctor to order a full thyroid panel. This will show the nuances and subtleties of your thyroid hormones and their interrelationships. Most people over age 50 respond very well to conventional thyroid treatment.

14

What Do You Do If You Want to Stop Treatment?

If you have thyroid imbalance, treatment is an inevitable consideration. The choices and decisions you make can have other health consequences. The idea of taking a pill every day for the rest of your life, as is currently conventional medicine's approach to hypothyroidism, might not appeal to you. You might not like the potential side effects of taking antithyroid drugs for hyperthyroidism, even though this is a time-limited treatment. But you can't opt out of treatment without jeopardizing your health. Although lifestyle factors strongly influence thyroid function (as well as other dimensions of your health), they are not enough to keep your thyroid in balance, and the consequences of unmanaged thyroid imbalance can be severe.

TREATMENT DECISIONS AND CONSEQUENCES: HYPERTHYROIDISM

Most people find the symptoms of hyperthyroidism unpleasant enough that the only question is which treatment is the best option. (See Chapter 11 for a full discussion of the treatment approaches for hyperthyroidism.) The consequences of opting for no treatment are immediate and even more unpleasant than the symptoms. Your body can't function at warp speed, as hyperthyroidism causes it to do, for very long before something gives. That could be your heart, your brain (stroke due to high blood pressure), your eyes—even your life itself. Health experts across disciplines—conventional as well as complementary—agree that medical treatment to control overactive thyroid is essential for health.

One life-threatening consequence of undetected or untreated hyperthyroidism is thyroid storm. When thyroid storm occurs, thyroid hormone suddenly floods your body. Cells react frantically to accommodate the influx by doing all that they are programmed to do—primarily boost metabolism—but instead send your body into chaos. Typically body temperature shoots up as high as 106°F and your heart rate becomes rapid, weak, and irregular. For a short time, perhaps several hours, you might experience wide mood swings, strong anxiety, and even psychosis. Thyroid storm typically progresses to coma, and, if not treated with emergency response to shut down thyroid function and stabilize heart function, can end in death. Usually some kind of stress to your body, such as illness or surgery, precipitates thyroid storm. Recovery with treatment is usually quick, with no lingering effects. The longer hyperthyroidism remains untreated, the more likely it is that you will experience thyroid storm.

HYPERTHYROIDISM AND HEART PROBLEMS

Overactive thyroid has both direct and indirect effects on your cardiovascular system—your heart and blood vessels. Untreated hyperthyroidism can:

- Elevate systolic blood pressure
- Intensify contractions that send blood from the heart more forcefully and with greater volume (increased cardiac output)

- Cause a change in the protein composition of heart muscle tissue that results in increased heart weight (cardiac hypertrophy)
- Alter the calcium and potassium levels of heart tissue, causing irregularities in heart rhythm (atrial fibrillation)
- Influence the adrenal glands to release cortisol and epinephrine, increasing heart rate (palpitations and ventricular tachycardia)
- Alter the heart's responses to nerve cell electrical impulses

Treatment to restore thyroid balance eliminates these changes and restores normal heart function. However, if any of these changes have persisted long enough to cause damage to the heart and blood vessels (or to the brain if they've caused a stroke), that damage is permanent.

HEART RHYTHM IRREGULARITIES

Hyperthyroidism causes three kinds of heart rhythm irregularities:

- Atrial fibrillation
- Ventricular tachycardia
- Atypical sinus rhythm

Atrial fibrillation is the most common of these irregularities, and can be the most insidious because you don't always feel that it is happening. When the heart is functioning normally, there is a close coordination between the two upper chambers of the heart (the atria), and the two lower chambers of the heart (the ventricles). Generally speaking, the atria receive blood and the ventricles send it out. The "DUB-dub" of your heartbeat reflects the strength of these respective rhythms: the pronounced "DUB" is the ventricular force, and the softer "dub" is the atrial force.

In atrial fibrillation, the atria beat much faster than the ventricles, and often without a consistent rhythm. You might feel this as mild palpitations, although most people don't feel it at all. The main consequence of this is that the ventricles then don't fill completely with blood; when it's their turn to contract, they expel their contents, but it isn't as much as it should be. This reduces the amount of blood—and the oxygen it carries—that your heart sends out into your body. Your cells signal that they're not happy with this, and your adrenal glands send cortisol and epinephrine to stimulate your heart to beat faster and harder. This increases the force of each ventricular beat, which compensates for the reduced blood volume . . . for a while.

Ventricular tachycardia (which means "rapid heartbeat") occurs when the ventricles, your heart's powerhouse pumping chambers, develop a fast, irregular rhythm. You almost always feel this as palpitations—the feeling that your pounding heart is about to explode from your chest. Ventricular tachycardia generally occurs in bursts that last a few seconds to a minute or so. When ventricular tachycardia occurs, your body rushes a number of remedial actions into place to end it quickly—if it were to continue, it would overtax your heart and cause a heart attack.

Atypical sinus rhythm (also called sinus tachycardia) occurs when the structure known as the sinoatrial node—your heart's natural pacemaker—becomes affected. This can happen for a number of reasons. One is the effect that elevated thyroid levels have on the action of calcium and potassium, the neuroconductors that transmit electrical impulses through the fibers of the heart, telling them when to contract and relax. Too much or too little of either of these electrolytes disturbs the intricate balance of these signals. Also, the adrenal gland's release of cortisol and epinephrine (the stress response) acts on the sinoatrial node. Increased sinus rhythm is also the body's response to increases in the rate of cellular metabolism, and sometimes accompanies a rise in body temperature. You might feel sinus tachycardia as a fast but regular heartbeat.

All of these irregularities, and the complicating heart problems they can cause, contribute to inadequate oxygenation—your heart can't get enough oxygen-bearing blood into your system. This of course further affects metabolism, because now your cells lack one of the source substances they need to complete their energy processes.

The increased levels of T3 circulating in your blood set up these irregularities by increasing heart cell metabolism and by activating the adrenal response. The further out of balance your thyroid function is, the more pronounced these irregularities become. Over time, they put great strain on the heart, causing it to enlarge in an effort to reduce its load. But the opposite effect usually occurs, with the heart's action becoming less efficient. This sets up a cycle of cardiac dysfunction that can result in life-threatening cardiac myopathy (a rare condition in which the heart enlarges to a point at which it is so tight in your chest that it can't pump) or in congestive heart failure (the heart becomes very inefficient).

Treatment to restore thyroid balance ends all of these changes. If they have become severe, your doctor might also prescribe drugs to treat the symptoms until your thyroid balance returns to normal. However, if any damage has occurred because of these changes, that damage is permanent.

High Blood Pressure

T3 acts on the cells in the smallest of your body's arteries, the arterioles, to cause these blood vessels to relax. This changes the force against which your heart is pumping to get blood out to these end-point arteries. In response, your body's endocrine matrix kicks into action, releasing hormones to raise your blood pressure to make sure your blood reaches its destination. The action is strongest for raising your systolic blood pressure, the pressure at the point of ventricular contraction. By itself, high blood pressure poses a variety of health risks. In combination with other heart function changes such as rhythm disturbances and compensatory responses by the heart—particularly increased cardiac output—the outcome can be deadly.

The risks of untreated high blood pressure are numerous and potentially serious, and include:

- Stroke
- Heart attack
- Coronary artery disease
- Kidney damage and kidney failure
- Damage to the retina of the eye and to the optic nerve
- Damage to peripheral blood vessels

High blood pressure, or hypertension as it's known by clinical diagnosis, is the leading cause of stroke and kidney failure. High blood pressure is especially dangerous when you also have diabetes (another autoimmune disorder), because the two conditions contribute to many of the same health problems.

If your high blood pressure is solely the result of thyroid imbalance, it will go away when your thyroid function returns to normal. High blood pressure has many causes, however, and becomes more common with increasing age. It is possible for high blood pressure to continue even after you restore your thyroid balance, and may require medication to lower it. Lifestyle factors such as body weight, diet, and physical activity also affect high blood pressure.

HEART ATTACK AND STROKE

Either untreated high blood pressure or persistent arrhythmias can cause heart attack. High blood pressure can cause tissue fragments or blood clots to break free from the walls of the arteries and lodge in the coronary arteries. This blocks the heart's blood supply, killing heart tissue and causing the affected part of the heart to stop functioning. High blood pressure can exploit any weakness in a coronary artery's wall, causing the area to split or rupture. The effect is the same: no blood supply to a portion of your heart. The location and extent of the damage determines how much effect there is on heart function.

Recovery from heart attack or stroke is independent of treatment for hyperthyroidism. Rapid medical treatment, including heart surgery if appropriate, and immediate rehabilitation for stroke, can minimize the long-term consequences of either health crisis. Treating overactive thyroid to restore balance can end the influence of thyroid hormone on blood pressure and heart rhythm.

HYPERTHYROIDISM AND OSTEOPOROSIS

Osteoporosis literally means "hollow bones." It is a condition that develops when bone tissue loses calcium, which results in lost bone mass and bone density. Thyroid hormones play an integral role in bone tissue activity. Because hyperthyroidism puts higher levels of thyroid hormone into the bloodstream, it increases calcium transfer.

Although osteoporosis is a more significant risk for women than for men, men experience bone loss with untreated hyperthyroidism, too. But because a man's bone density and mass are higher than a woman's to begin with, it takes longer for the loss to cause problems or symptoms.

THE REMODELING CYCLE

Although we think of bone as hard and inert, it's actually just as active as any cellular structure in your body. Your body is continually forming new bone cells and destroying old bone cells. This keeps your bones healthy and strong. Medically, this is known as remodeling, and it is a continuous process that takes place in bone tissue throughout your body. Remodeling is most active along the surface of bones, and takes place in multiple but noncontiguous segments along the bone's surface. These are called activation sites.

Two kinds of bone cells participate in remodeling, osteoclasts and osteoblasts. Osteoclasts act first. They are the "destroyers"; osteoclast means "to break bone." They resorb, or consume, bone cells that have reached the end of their useful lives. Osteoblasts act next. They are the "builders"; osteoblast means "to germinate bone." When your body is in balance, each remodeling cycle takes about 200 days. Thousands of cycles are taking place, starting and ending at different times.

A number of factors affect the remodeling cycle, one of which is thyroid hormone. Thyroid hormone stimulates the activation of a remodeling cycle. The more thyroid hormone that is in the bloodstream and reaches bone cells, the more cycles it stimulates. As the number of remodeling cycles increases, the less bone surface is available for new cycles to start. To compensate, remodeling cycles shorten. Although both phases shorten equally—resorption and formation—formation takes the greater hit. The reason for this lies deep within the cells, in those busy engines of cell activity, the mitochondria.

Osteoblast mitochondria have T3 receptors, allowing direct T3 binding (Chapter 3 discusses these processes). Because of this, they respond more rapidly to the effects of available thyroid hormone. Hyperthyroidism elevates T3 levels, both by increasing T4 and T3 production and by increasing T4-to-T3 conversion. More available T3 allows more T3 mitochondrial binding, which in turn increases mitochondrial and cell metabolism.

Osteoclast mitochondria do not have T3 receptors, so T3 affects them indirectly. Eventually their metabolism also increases, but lags behind the increased metabolism of osteoblasts. The result is an imbalance in the remodeling cycle that causes bone tissue to be lost faster than it is replaced. The difference can result in bone loss of 2 percent to 5 percent a month, which can lead to seriously weakened bone structure within a year or less. All too often, unfortunately, the first sign of any problem is spontaneous fracture—a break in the bone that happens without apparent cause.

Calcium Depletion

Another component of the bone weakening that occurs with osteoporosis is calcium depletion. Calcium is a fundamental building block of bone tissue. It is also essential for many body functions, particularly transmitting the electrical signals of nerve cell communication. The signals that coordinate heart function, for example, depend on appropriate calcium levels. Your bones are your body's warehouses for storing calcium.

When calcium levels in your bloodstream drop, various hormones activate a sequence of events that allow your body to draw calcium out of your bones to boost blood levels back up. These hormones include parathyroid hormone (PTH) and the "other" thyroid hormone, calcitonin. (Although hyperthyroidism doesn't directly affect calcitonin production, the interrelationships of hormone balance within the endocrine matrix come into play.) This withdrawal further exacerbates bone weakness.

Cutting the Losses

Calcium supplements and "impact" exercise are the most effective approaches to preventing bone tissue loss both for women and for men. Calcium supplements give your body extra calcium supplies to meet its everyday needs, so it doesn't need to extract calcium from your bones. Although calcium is the most critical, it is not the only nutrient necessary for bone formation. Vitamin D, which comes from natural sunlight and from certain foods, enables your body to properly absorb and use calcium. Magnesium, boron, vitamin K, and B vitamins are also part of bone metabolism.

Impact exercise, such as walking or running, stimulates osteoblast activity to produce new growth in bone tissue, helping to strengthen bone structure. Once bone tissue is lost, it's difficult to replace it. Raising calcium intake helps strengthen remaining bone tissue, but can't create new bone. New drugs, such as Fosamax, are able to restore some of bone tissue lost to osteoporosis, but not all of it.

Bone loss in women also is linked to estrogen levels; a woman's risk for osteoporosis dramatically increases with menopause, when estrogen levels decline. Accordingly, most treatments target keeping estrogen levels up. Since osteoporosis becomes a significant health risk after menopause, conventional hormone replacement therapy (HRT) has long been the treatment of choice for prevention.

With HRT, a woman takes supplemental estrogen and progestin in cyclical doses to mimic, on a lower level of function, the monthly ebb and flow of these hormones that characterized her fertility before menopause. The hormone levels are lower than during her fertile years, so they don't restore fertility. But they are high enough to support healthy bone calcium levels.

In recent years, however, HRT has come under scrutiny and challenge. Some studies suggest that HRT lessens bone loss and the severity of osteoporosis, they also raise concerns about health problems that HRT can cause. The most disturbing is the link between estrogen and certain kinds of breast and uterine cancers. Drugs called selective estrogen receptor modulators, or SERMs, are getting much attention for their ability to influence bone stability without affecting other estrogen-sensitive processes (more about this in Chapter 18).

All the supportive treatments modern medicine can offer, however, are like pouring water into a leaking bucket. They can keep trying to maintain bone mass and density, but your over-active thyroid continues to drain their effectiveness. Unless you restore the balance of thyroid activity and hormone in your body, osteoporosis will remain a challenge to your health.

HYPERTHYROIDISM AND FERTILITY PROBLEMS

Overactive thyroid can suppress a woman's menstrual cycle through its effect on sex hormones and on cell metabolism (see Chapter 18). Through the delicate interplay among components of your endocrine matrix, increased thyroid hormone stimulates a cascade of events that results in elevated estrogen and testosterone levels. This affects the levels of follicle-stimulating hormone (FSH), which directs egg development, and luteinizing hormone (LH), which regulates egg maturity and release.

In a normal menstrual cycle, estrogen levels drop and progesterone levels rise following ovulation, to prepare the uterus for receiving a fertilized egg should there be one. If there isn't, the extra tissue and blood that has carpeted the uterine wall sloughs away as menstrual flow, and the cycle starts anew. In a menstrual cycle under the influence of hyperthyroidism, estrogen levels also drop, but because they are high to start with they don't reach the same valley level as during normal cycling. This inhibits progesterone to some extent, and the thickening of the uterine wall is much lighter than normal.

This sequence of events affects fertility in two ways. First, the disturbances to FSH and LH interfere with egg development, maturation, and release. If your ovaries don't release an egg at midcycle, you cannot conceive. Second, the limited preparation of the uterus discourages implantation. Even if you did release an egg and it became fertilized, it would have trouble lodging in the uterus.

In men, hyperthyroidism increases testosterone levels, which accelerates sperm maturation. This can result in releasing sperm that are not yet mature, and so are incapable of fertilization.

Fertility that is solely the consequence of thyroid imbalance returns to normal once thyroid function does. Your doctor might discover that you have overactive thyroid during examination for fertility problems, especially if your hyperthyroidism is in its early stages or is low-grade. Fertility is another delicate and complex balance within your body, and many factors in addition to thyroid balance influence it. Hypothyroidism also affects fertility, but in different ways—more about that later in this chapter.

HYPERTHYROIDISM AND EYE PROBLEMS

One of the most distressing symptoms of hyperthyroidism is exophthalmos, or bulging eyes. This problem is unique to Graves' disease and arises when the autoimmune response of this condition affects the tissues of the eye and the muscles that control the eye. It's known clinically as infiltrative ophthalmopathy, a reference to the infiltration by lymph cells into the tissues of and surrounding the eyes. Although infiltrative ophthalmopathy begins as a consequence of Graves' disease, once under way it becomes a separate condition. Treating the underlying hyperthyroidism helps to end the autoimmune response that's attacking the structures of the eye, but it doesn't reverse any of the damage.

As well, infiltrative ophthalmopathy can continue on its own path, separate from the course of your hyperthyroidism. This requires the attention of an ophthalmologist (physician who specializes in care of the eyes). This is the most important reason to seek prompt medical treatment at the earliest signs of eye involvement, which typically include:

- Bulging eyes
- The appearance of a fixed stare
- Droopy eyelids or eyelids that appear pulled back

- Red, irritated eyes and excessive tearing
- Pain around the eyes (orbital pain)
- Sensitivity to light and pain with exposure to light (photophobia)
- Double vision

Sometimes mild eye symptoms appear with forms of hyper-thyroidism other than Graves' disease. These do go away with treatment to restore thyroid balance. Infiltrative ophthalmopathy can appear before or after Graves' disease (even by years).

HYPERTHYROIDISM AND SKIN PROBLEMS

Sometimes in Graves' disease there is also lymph infiltration into the tissues of the skin along the tops of the shins. It's not clear why this infiltration locates here. The condition is known clinically as infiltrative dermopathy (sometimes called pretibial myxedema). It starts with a red, itchy rash. As the rash heals, it forms into leatherlike patches that are somewhat tawny in color.

Infiltrative dermopathy is usually the second part of a double whammy—it tends to accompany infiltrative ophthalmopathy. And like its ophthalmic counterpart, once it emerges, infiltrative dermopathy runs its own course independent of hyperthyroidism, and can appear before or after Graves' disease shows up. Topical medications such as those used to treat eczema can help relieve the symptoms.

TREATMENT DECISIONS AND CONSEQUENCES: HYPOTHYROIDISM

Because hypothyroidism typically develops over a long period of time—years and even decades—it's easy to conclude that underactive thyroid is more of a nuisance than a health problem with potentially serious consequences. But hypothyroidism is insidious. If you've had symptoms for some time before seeing a doctor about them, chances are you're already experiencing some health consequences. Although some of them, such as the accumulation of arterial plaque as a result of elevated blood cholesterol, can be permanent or might require additional treatment, most of them reverse when your thyroid balance returns to normal.

Underactive thyroid in which you have symptoms, but blood thyroid levels are within a normal range, is most likely to respond to alternative approaches to controlling your symptoms, such as through diet and lifestyle. Even so, it's important to have blood thyroid tests at least once a year so you can keep track of whether the imbalance is worsening. If your symptoms continue or get worse after you've tried other methods for three months or so, it's time to reconsider your treatment options.

A potentially life-threatening consequence of untreated hypothyroidism is myxedemic coma. Like its hyperthyroid counterpart, thyroid storm, myxedemic coma comes on suddenly and with little warning. Feelings of being cold and drowsy rapidly progress to seizures and coma, often within just a few hours. Body temperature plummets to critical levels as thyroid function virtually ceases, leaving cells with no fuel source for the activities of metabolism. Your body goes into a state of shock, shutting down nonessential systems first and then even essential systems in an attempt to regain control.

Emergency treatment requires intravenous thyroid hormone to restart cell metabolism, and often drugs to boost heart rate and respiration back to functional levels. Recovery is usually complete and without lasting consequences. Typically some sort of physical stress, such as illness or surgery, sets off the sequence of events that culminate in myxedemic coma. Without medical treatment to supply your body with thyroid hormone, you remain vulnerable to further episodes.

HYPOTHYROIDISM AND HEART DISEASE

Some health experts consider underactive thyroid to be one of the leading contributors to heart disease, although it gets little mention for its role. T3 and T4 are essential players in your body's processing of lipids and fatty acids. Low thyroid function nearly always means high blood cholesterol, and it doesn't take long for high blood cholesterol to become coronary artery disease.

HIGH BLOOD CHOLESTEROL

The body gets rid of cholesterol by emulsifying it in bile from the liver and gall bladder, converting it to bile salts. This occurs in the inner mitochondrial membrane. For cholesterol to come into the mitochondrial membrane, it needs a transport protein that in turn needs T3 in order to work. T3 also activates bile salts from the hepatocytes. Thus thyroid dysfunction can lead to both increased risk of heart disease and of gall bladder disease, both relating to the inability to convert cholesterol to bile salts. T3 increases boost the genetic expression of the LDL receptor gene, leading to increased receptor activity and therefore less LDL available.

High blood cholesterol contributes to coronary heart disease, and also can result in stroke or heart attack if pieces of arterial plaque break free from the arterial walls and lodge in the brain or the heart. Lowering blood cholesterol, especially LDL, decreases the severity of coronary artery disease. Restoring thyroid balance alone is not always enough to improve blood cholesterol levels if significant arterial plaque accumulations have taken place. Other medications might be necessary to return blood cholesterol to healthy levels (see Chapter 17).

CORONARY ARTERY DISEASE

Because of its role in allowing high blood cholesterol to develop, hypothyroidism is an indirect but key cause of coronary artery disease. Coronary artery disease exists when the arteries that supply the heart itself with blood become blocked or narrowed to the extent that the damage impedes the flow of blood. Less blood means less oxygen makes it to the heart tissues, resulting in a condition called ischemia (a word of Greek origin that means "to hold back blood").

Oddly enough, underactive thyroid can minimize the effects that coronary artery disease has on the heart. Lower blood levels of T3 and T4, of course, decrease cell metabolism. When this occurs in the cells of the heart, it reduces their need for oxygen as well. This makes the situation of diminished blood flow less of a problem. Restoring thyroid balance can, in fact, cause angina to flare up—pain related to insufficient oxygen to the heart.

So does it help ischemia to leave hypothyroidism untreated? In the short term, perhaps, but in the long term it causes even more problems as the coronary artery disease responsible for the ischemia worsens. Eventually your heart will reach a point at which it's not getting enough blood and oxygen to meet even its diminished needs, and it will let you know this. You might experience a flare-up of angina . . . or a heart attack (myocardial infarction) when the oxygen level gets low enough to cause heart tissue to die.

High Blood Pressure

Initially, underactive thyroid results in low blood pressure. As your metabolism slows, so does your body's need for the nutrients (including oxygen) that your blood distributes. Since cells are receiving adequate nourishment, the intricate network of biochemical signals lets your heart know it doesn't need to pump quite so hard or efficiently. Blood pressure drops.

If this was the last link in the chain of events, we might consider induced hypothyroidism as treatment for high blood pressure! But of course we don't, because it's not. All that cholesterol that's accumulating in your arteries is narrowing and stiffening them, causing a condition called atherosclerosis. This gives your arteries increased resistance, so even though the demand for oxygen and other nutrients is down, your heart has to work harder to get blood through your arteries. In the end, the result is *high* blood pressure.

Your blood pressure may or may not return to normal if you restore thyroid balance. The degree of atherosclerosis that is present becomes more important than the direct effects of thyroid hormone. It is possible that even when your thyroid functions return to normal, your blood pressure will remain elevated, requiring medical treatment. Untreated high blood pressure has numerous and potentially serious health consequences, as we discussed earlier in this chapter.

HYPOTHYROIDISM AND OSTEOPOROSIS

Underactive thyroid itself seems to have no effect on the remodeling cycle of bone tissue destruction and construction. However, getting too much thyroid hormone supplement can have the same effect as being hyperthyroid.

CHOOSING TO GO WITHOUT TREATMENT: DOING BATTLE WITH YOUR OWN BODY

One of the major factors in the enormous increase of autoimmune problems in the past thirty to forty years is environmental in nature. What else is autoimmunity, if not the result of a constant bombardment of our immune systems until they become hyper-reactive? Clearly there are genetic factors, but this doesn't explain at all the individual variability in gene expression and so on. Autoimmune illnesses, and in fact most illnesses, are the result of the internal and external environment playing out through the moment-to-moment unique expression of individual genes.

Those genes are, in turn, subject to occasional mutations (sometimes called "single nucleotide polymorphisms" or SniPs), which are themselves the result of environmental conditions, and appear to give us all of our individual characteristics from eye color to metabolic defects to the tendency toward run-on sentences! This is a critical point of the metabolic matrix, the fact that there is a constant interplay between the internal and external environments, playing out through moment-to-moment gene expression.

The odds are against you when you choose to forgo treatment for thyroid imbalance. For a short time, you might be able to create an environment of balance through lifestyle actions, primarily diet and perhaps nutritional supplements. All health experts recommend that medical treatment be a part of managing thyroid balance. Lifestyle actions can support this treatment, and even minimize the extent to which you need it. But they can't replace it. Leaving thyroid imbalance untreated has serious health consequences. For the most part, when you have symptoms, your thyroid imbalance has reached the point at which the other components of your endocrine matrix can no longer compensate. Continuing without treatment jeopardizes your health and your life.

Part 4

Restoring Thyroid Health: Living in Balance

15

Nutrition: Foods That Help, Foods That Don't Help

The foods you eat fuel your body's needs. Some foods help restore and maintain thyroid balance, while other foods undermine your efforts to correct either overactive or underactive thyroid. We are only now beginning to understand the intricate and complex role that foods play at every level of metabolism.

YOUR THYROID GLAND'S DIETARY NEEDS: IODINE AND TYROSINE

Your thyroid gland needs two substances from your diet: iodine and tyrosine. These are the substances it uses to make thyroid hormones (T3 and T4). It doesn't take that much of either to meet your thyroid's needs, but consuming inadequate amounts of either can significantly alter your thyroid balance. If one or the other ingredient is missing, then your thyroid can't make enough thyroid hormone, and hypothyroidism results. And too much of both ingredients produces the opposite result, hyperthyroidism.

IODINE

Iodine is an element found in a number of food sources. Lack of iodine is the leading cause of thyroid dysfunction throughout the world, although it is seldom a contributing factor in developed countries such as those in North America and Western Europe. Because the most significant natural source of iodine is seawater, the further you live from the ocean (or where oceans once were), the more likely it is that natural sources of iodine are limited. Iodine remains in the soil, and is absorbed by grains, vegetables, and fruits that grow in it. In the United States, regions along the Great Lakes and through the central plains have the lowest levels of naturally occurring iodine.

Your thyroid gland is the only tissue in your body that absorbs or uses iodine. Whatever iodine your thyroid cannot absorb, your body excretes through your urine. When evaluating the thyroid's ability to use iodine, doctors sometimes test the urine for iodine content.

FOOD SOURCES OF IODINE

Many foods contain at least trace amounts of iodine, particularly those that come from the sea or are grown in iodine-rich soil. Common foods that are high in iodine include:

- Shellfish such as shrimp (prawns) and lobster
- Ocean finfish such as tuna and salmon (fresh and canned)
- Kelp, dulse, and other edible kinds of seaweed
- Onions
- Asparagus
- Dairy products, particularly milk
- Processed foods such as baked goods and fast-food items with high sodium content

The body's iodine need is miniscule—just 150 micrograms

a day, an amount equivalent to ½ teaspoonful of iodized salt. Most people can get all the iodine they need from eating foods high in iodine.

IODIZED SALT

Sea salt is naturally high in iodine. The processed table salt that most of us use is not. The process of refining salt removes iodine from it; iodized salt has had iodine added back to it. Some countries, such as Canada, require that all salt be iodized. In the United States, iodized salt is an option that about half of Americans use. In many other parts of the world, iodized salt is not available at all, although some countries add iodine to grains, dairy products, or drinking water to make sure people receive an adequate amount of dietary iodine.

Some baking processes add a different form of iodine, called iodates, to dough to make it more consistent and easier to work with. This is why baked goods, especially bread, tend to be high in iodine. Commercial baking processes also use large amounts of iodized salt, further increasing the iodine content of the finished product. Iodine is also a common disinfectant and antibacterial agent in cleaning solutions used to clean food-processing equipment and milking and dairy equipment. The residue of such cleaners can leach into milk and other foods.

Because vegetable sources are so unpredictable as sources of iodine, most people benefit from using iodized salt to make sure they receive enough iodine. If you eat a lot of fish, shellfish, and other foods high in iodine, you can probably choose to use non-iodized salt without jeopardizing your thyroid health. If you're uncertain about the iodine levels of the foods you eat, or know that you don't eat many iodine-rich foods, iodized salt is a safe and effective source of iodine. For most people the greater health risk is actually from too much salt, which is linked to medical problems such as high blood pressure, rather than too much iodine.

Too Much of a Good Thing

Too much iodine is poisonous and can permanently damage the thyroid gland. Too much iodine during pregnancy can totally suppress development of the thyroid gland in the fetus. The toxic level for iodine is 1 milligram (1,000 micrograms), which is about seven times the recommended daily allowance. Early symptoms of iodine poisoning are the same as for overactive thyroid, and the two are often inseparable because too much iodine causes hyperthyroidism.

TYROSINE

Tyrosine is a conditionally essential amino acid that your body forms from the metabolism of the essential amino acid phenylalanine. Essential amino acids are those that you must supply to your body through dietary sources, usually proteins. Nonessential amino acids are those that your body makes from other substances. And conditionally essential amino acids are those that your body might become unable to manufacture, making it necessary for you to supply them through the foods you eat.

Tyrosine affects a number of points within your endocrine matrix:

- Your pituitary gland uses tyrosine to manufacture melanocyte-stimulating hormone, which is responsible for darkening skin pigmentation in response to sun exposure.
- Your adrenal glands use tyrosine to make the neurotransmitter norepinephrine, which acts on certain areas of your brain that affect your mood. A shortage of norepinephrine can cause, among other problems, depression.
- Your adrenal glands and a part of your brain called the substantia nigra use tyrosine to make another neurotransmitter, dopamine. Dopamine has a number of functions, one of which is to permit normal skeletal muscle movements.

Dopamine depletion is a hallmark of Parkinson's disease, in which nerve signals to muscle cells become jumbled. The anti-Parkinson's drug levodopa is manufactured from tyrosine. And researchers are exploring whether tyrosine supplementation might offset the tremors and stiff movements that characterize this debilitating condition. Recent research suggests that dopamine plays a role in our choosing "natural rewards" such as food and love over "unnatural rewards" like addictions and risky behaviors.

- And of course, your thyroid gland uses tyrosine, combined with iodine, to produce the thyroid hormones, primarily T3 and T4.

FOOD SOURCES OF TYROSINE

Your body makes most of the tyrosine it needs when it metabolizes the essential amino acid phenylalanine. However, some foods contain small amounts of tyrosine. These include:

- Soybeans and food products made from them
- Chicken and other poultry
- Fish
- Almonds, pumpkin seeds, and sesame seeds
- Avocados
- Bananas
- Lima beans and other legumes
- Dairy products

There are also many nutritional supplement products that contain tyrosine. These products typically claim to improve memory, mood, energy level, sex drive (libido), and thyroid health. Anecdotal research tends to support these claims, although scientific evidence is incomplete.

Because the body manufactures most of the tyrosine it needs from phenylalanine, the most efficient sources of tyrosine are foods that contain phenylalanine. Any food that is considered a complete protein contains all of the essential amino acids that the human body requires, including phenylalanine. These foods include:

- Meat
- Fish
- Poultry
- Eggs
- Milk
- Aspartame (the artificial sweetener)

Many people have trouble digesting protein, which can lead to decreased body levels of amino acids including tyrosine and phenylalanine. Some people have a genetic metabolic disorder, phenylketonuria (PKU), that prevents their bodies from converting phenylalanine into tyrosine. Without intervention, this disorder allows phenylalanine to accumulate in the body, causing irreparable harm to brain tissue. Treatment is to avoid dietary phenylalanine, which means following a lifelong, strict vegetarian diet (avoiding all animal sources of protein). Because by the time symptoms show up it's usually too late to prevent neurological damage, hospitals in the United States routinely test all newborns for PKU. People with PKU often have hypothyroidism, because they are not getting enough tyrosine (via phenylalanine) for their thyroid glands to make adequate amounts of thyroid hormone.

IODINE + TYROSINE = THYROID HORMONE

Here are the technical details of how iodine and tyrosine combine to become thyroid hormones. During digestion, dietary iodine converts to an atomic, or free elemental, form called iodide. In this form, iodide is able to attach to protein molecules that then carry it to your thyroid gland.

Tyrosine enters your digestive system in the form of protein. Digestion converts this protein into its basic components, amino acids. These amino acids—including phenylalanine, which becomes converted tyrosine—and small amounts of tyrosine itself enter your bloodstream. As your blood carries the tyrosine molecules through your thyroid gland, your thyroid tissues extract what they need.

Inside the tissues of your thyroid gland, iodide combines with oxygen and tyrosine. The resulting product is either monoiodotyrosine (MIT), which has a single iodide atom, or diiodotyrosine (DIT), which has two iodide atoms. In these forms, these substances are usually considered inactive hormones, although recent research supports a metabolic active role for DIT. MIT and DIT then further combine to form either T3 or T4, becoming active hormones. A MIT plus a DIT becomes T3 (three iodide atoms). A DIT plus a DIT becomes T4 (four iodide atoms). Your thyroid gland then stores T3 and T4 until it needs to send it out to the cells in your body. In the liver and peripheral cells, an iodine atom is then removed from T4, creating either T3 or reverse T3 (rT3).

THYROID-SUPRESSING FOODS

Some foods contain enzymes called thiocyanates, which act like antithyroid drugs. They interfere with your thyroid gland's ability to take in iodine, which in turn limits its ability to produce thyroid hormone. Sometimes these foods are called goitrogenic, or "goiter-growing." In theory, goitrogenic foods could suppress thyroid hormone production to the extent that a goiter forms. This is not very likely in today's society, however. The greater risk from eating large quantities of thyroid-suppressing foods is that they more subtly affect thyroid function.

One group of compounds, called flavonoids, are responsible for the sweet smells, pleasant tastes, and bright colors of fruits and vegetables. Many flavonoids resemble the T4 molecule, and can interfere with its function, leading to suppressing of thyroid function. Although this effect is unlikely in the amounts of fruits and vegetables eaten by most people, it becomes important when you are taking supplements containing bioflavonoids, particularly one flavonoid supplement called quercitin, which is used to treat allergy.

Common thyroid-suppressing foods include:

- Cruciferous vegetables such as cauliflower, broccoli, kale, brussels sprouts, and cabbage
- Rutabagas, turnips, radishes, carrots
- Peaches, strawberries
- Peanuts
- Spinach
- Watercress
- Soybeans and food products high in soy isoflavones

Cooking seems to reduce the thyroid-suppressing effect of cruciferous vegetables, carrots, and spinach. However, cooking also decreases or destroys many nutrients that these vegetables contain when you eat them raw.

Many of these foods—in particular soy isoflavones and cruciferous vegetables—have valuable anticancer qualities. They also influence other hormone levels, such as estrogen and progesterone in women and testosterone in men. Carrots are an excellent dietary source of beta carotene, which your body converts into vitamin A. And all of these foods are high in dietary fiber, making them good choices for digestive health. Do you have to give up these foods—and their health benefits—when you have thyroid imbalance?

ARE THYROID-SUPRESSING FOODS AFFECTING YOUR THYROID BALANCE?

Whether foods could be affecting your thyroid balance depends on whether your thyroid treatment seems effective, an assessment that needs to include both lab values and your symptoms. Eating thyroid-suppressing foods in moderate amounts isn't likely to affect your thyroid function. But a diet high in these foods can interfere with, minimize, or even cancel out the effect of thyroid hormone supplement to treat underactive thyroid, and is sometimes the culprit when treatment doesn't appear to work.

If you're taking thyroid hormone supplement but still have symptoms of underactive thyroid, keep a food journal for a week. Write down everything that you eat, how much of it you eat, and in what combinations you usually eat it. At the end of a week, analyze your eating habits. Are most of the fruits and vegetables that you eat thyroid-suppressing? If so, ask your doctor to test your blood thyroid levels.

Then reduce (not necessarily eliminate) the amounts of these foods you eat for two weeks. Again, write down what and how much you eat, so you know for certain what you're actually consuming. Ask your doctor to retest your blood thyroid levels. Is there a difference, however slight? How do you feel? If there is a perceptible change in your blood levels and you feel better, then you've probably been overdoing it with the thyroid-suppressing foods (and most likely haven't known you were, since not all doctors know of the connection between these foods and thyroid balance).

It is possible for thyroid function to return to normal once you reduce your consumption of thyroid-suppressing foods, if you were indeed eating enough of them to cause problems. Usually the process of reduction will make it clear whether this is the case for you. It's not particularly common for goitrogenic foods to be blamed, but it can be the case if your consumption of these foods was very high and you have continued to experience symptoms of underactive thyroid even after starting thyroid hormone treatment. Have your blood thyroid levels checked regularly, however, to make sure your thyroid balance really is restored.

CAN THYROID-SUPPRESSING FOODS IMPROVE OVERACTIVE THYROID?

Most doctors are reluctant to use foods to treat overactive thyroid because the consequences of inadequate treatment can be serious. However, if you have had conventional treatment for overactive thyroid and are no longer taking antithyroid drugs, eating moderate to high amounts of thyroid-suppressing foods might help keep your thyroid gland from again becoming overactive.

It remains important to have regular thyroid blood tests and to pay attention to early symptoms of either overactive or underactive thyroid. About half of people who undergo treatment for overactive thyroid eventually become hypothyroid. If you're eating a lot of thyroid-suppressing foods to stave off another bout of hyperthyroidism, you could end up accelerating your transition to underactive thyroid.

SOY AND SOY FOOD PRODUCTS

Soy supplements have become a mainstay of complementary therapy for women for problems related to premenstrual syndrome (PMS) and menopause, and to help prevent breast and uterine cancers. Soy foods, soy supplements, and cruciferous vegetables have shown significant promise in preventing and delaying the spread of prostate cancer in men. However, there has been some research that suggests that a diet high in isoflavones, and particularly genistein, also suppresses thyroid function, causing hypothyroidism. Some studies have detected higher-than-average rates of hypothyroidism in adults who were fed soy-based formulas as infants.

Although these findings are far from conclusive and involve people who were ingesting large amounts of isoflavones, they do raise the specter of concern. If you have thyroid imbalance and you want to have a high dietary intake of soy and cruciferous vegetables for their many health benefits, make sure your doctor tests your blood thyroid levels regularly.

Pay close attention to how you feel and whether you seem to be developing symptoms of underactive thyroid. If it appears that you are, ease off these foods a bit and see what difference it makes. Most of the time you won't need to give up these foods entirely, but you might need to cut back on them to maintain thyroid balance.

Soy food products that might affect thyroid function include:

- Soymilk
- Soy nut butter
- Roasted or boiled soybeans
- Tofu
- Tempeh
- Soy protein isolate (usually sold as a supplement in powder or capsule form)
- Textured soy protein

If you want to eat these foods, make sure that your iodine intake is adequate. Remember that with iodine, a little goes a long way, so don't overdo it. Just make sure that you reach the daily minimum of 150 micrograms, which is easy enough through dietary sources that are high in iodine, such as fish and milk.

MINERALS, VITAMINS, AND THYROID FUNCTION

Minerals can interfere with the absorption of many nutrients and medications. Calcium and iron both reduce the amount of thyroid hormone supplement that enters your bloodstream from your digestive tract. Many foods that are high in calcium are easy to identify: milk, cheese, and dairy products head the list. Others aren't so obvious, like tofu, canned sardines, molasses, spinach, broccoli, and green beans.

Because calcium has become such an important health concern for maintaining bone health, many food products are fortified with calcium. One of the most common of these is orange juice. Most people take their thyroid hormone supplement in the morning. If you are one of them, and you then have milk and orange juice with breakfast, you might end up canceling out much of the supplement's effect. Pop your daily multivitamin with iron and calcium, and you've certainly done so!

Take your thyroid hormone at least two hours before or after taking multivitamins or eating foods high in calcium. Most doctors and pharmacists recommend that you take thyroid hormone on an empty stomach, and then have nothing to eat or drink (other than water), for 30 minutes. This allows the supplement to get into your digestive tract without interference from food.

Other vitamins and minerals aid thyroid function. Beta carotene helps your thyroid gland produce thyroid hormone. In return, T3 is necessary for the your body to produce vitamin A from beta carotene. Some people develop a yellowish coloration on their palms and the soles of their feet if they are unable to convert the carotenes in their diet to active forms. This can be a subtle sign of thyroid deficiency.

Selenium is necessary for the de-iodinase enzyme that produces T3 from T4. Vitamin E protects thyroid hormone from being broken down. Vitamins B_2, B_6, C, and niacin also improve thyroid function. Zinc plays a key role in immune function and also cell health. And calcium, even though you need to take it separately from thyroid hormone supplement, is particularly important when thyroid imbalance is a factor, because thyroid function affects how your body uses and stores calcium.

These days, many people take nutritional products on the advice of friends, natural medicine doctors, even Internet chatrooms. It's important to know the effects of these products. Nutrients other than vitamins and minerals also influence thyroid function. If taken in high doses, L-carnitine, an amino acid used for energy, can suppress thyroid function by blocking T3 production. Alpha lipoic acid, a potent antioxidant, has a similar effect.

FIBER

It doesn't make much difference one way or the other, from the perspective of thyroid balance, whether your diet is high in fiber or low in fiber. What does matter is that it *stays* one way or the other. Fiber influences the way your intestines absorb nutrients. A diet high in fiber is known to help protect against a variety of digestive system conditions, including colon cancer. It also aids in limiting the amount of dietary fat that your intestine digests. The reason for this is that fiber acts to move things right along through your digestive tract. Nutrients that take a long time to digest—like dietary fats—don't get to stay long enough for complete digestion, and so pass from your body as waste.

The amount of fiber in your diet influences how your digestive system absorbs medications, too. Drugs that absorb through the intestine, like thyroid hormone supplement, are the most significantly affected. When you take thyroid hormone supplement, your doctor measures your blood hormone levels at certain intervals until those levels reach normal range and stay there. Your doctor might adjust your thyroid supplement dose several times to find the dose that produces the desired effect. Once you reach stability, this is the dose you continue to take.

Most people maintain fairly steady eating habits (which is partly why weight becomes a problem; more on this in Chapter

16). The amount of fiber in your diet isn't likely to change unless you decide to make a change in your eating habits. Say you're reading a book (even this book) and you decide that your eating habits aren't really supporting your health as they could and should. You, like many Americans, eat a diet high in carbohydrates and fats, and relatively skimpy on vegetables, fruits, and whole grains. So you decide to eat more of the latter and less of the former.

This is great for your overall health! But it is likely to affect your thyroid balance. Fruits, vegetables, and whole grains are the main sources of dietary fiber. If you go from barely any of these foods in your diet to eating them with every meal (which is what's most healthy for your body), your digestive balance changes. Odds are, before making this change you might have had bowel movements every two days or even less frequently. Suddenly you're having at least one bowel movement daily, and maybe two or three. This is your clue that your intestines are now working efficiently.

The fiber you've added through your dietary changes adds bulk to your intestinal contents. And added bulk stimulates peristalsis, the rhythmic waves of smooth muscle contraction that move this content through your digestive tract. It is this faster movement, in fact, that researchers believe accounts for fiber's role in lowering the risk of colon cancer: potential toxins spend far less time lingering where they could be absorbed into your tissues.

The increased speed with which food now makes its way through your digestive system means that drugs such as your thyroid hormone supplement don't linger as long, either. So less of the supplement makes it from the pill into your body. This has the effect of dropping your dosage level. If this level has been appropriate for balancing your thyroid function, it is now not enough. Gradually you will see the symptoms of underactive thyroid re-emerge. Don't change back to your old eating habits, though! Just let your doctor know that you want to have your blood levels retested.

Once you make a change to add more fiber to your diet, stick with it on a daily basis. Bouncing from lots of fiber to no fiber from day to day confuses your digestive system, making absorption of nutrients and medications alike inconsistent. Foods that are high in fiber include:

- Fruits such as apples, oranges, pineapple, strawberries
- Vegetables such as carrots, broccoli, cauliflower, cabbage, brussels sprouts
- Whole grains such as oats, barley, corn
- Legumes such as peas, lima beans, pinto beans, red beans
- Products made from whole grains, such as whole wheat or whole grain breads and cereals

Going from a diet high in fiber to one low in fiber also will affect how your body absorbs thyroid hormone supplement, although this change is not as common because the typical American diet is low in fiber. If you suddenly drop the fiber content of your diet, the amount of thyroid hormone supplement that your intestines absorb will increase. This could result in symptoms of overactive thyroid, as your blood thyroid levels would rise. For most people, it makes sense to return to a diet higher in fiber. But check with your doctor, and have your blood thyroid hormone levels checked to be sure you're taking the appropriate dose of thyroid supplement.

CHOOSING YOUR DIET TO HELP YOUR THYROID BALANCE

Nutritional balance supports every body function, and thyroid is no exception. From supplying the nutrients that your thyroid gland needs to make thyroid hormone to fueling the rest of your body's needs, the choices you make about the foods you eat affect your health. For most people, following the nutrition guidelines set forth by the U. S. Department of Agriculture (USDA) in the food pyramid and other sources is the most important action you can take for overall good health. If you are taking treatment for either underactive or overactive thyroid, choose foods to support thyroid balance.

For underactive thyroid:
- Limit the amount of goitrogenic foods (such as cruciferous vegetables) that you eat.
- Eat moderate amounts of foods that are high in iodine, such as fish.
- Eat enough protein to supply your body's tyrosine needs.
- Eat foods that supply B vitamins, vitamin C, vitamin E, and beta carotene (a form of vitamin A) and the minerals calcium, selenium, and zinc.

For overactive thyroid:
- Eat moderate amounts of raw cruciferous vegetables and other goitrogenic foods to help limit your thyroid's hormone production.
- Eat plenty of colorful and flavorful fruits and vegetables.
- Eat foods that are high in vitamin C.
- Eat adequate, but not excessive, amounts of foods that supply protein.

Nutrition is not a substitute for treatment when it comes to thyroid balance. But good eating habits can work in tandem with drug treatments to improve your thyroid health.

16

Keeping Your Weight in Balance

For several decades after the discovery of antithyroid therapy to treat hyperthyroidism in the 1940s, doctors tended to view persistent weight problems as glandular problems. The thyroid had clear responsibility for weight loss accompanying hyperthyroidism. Doctors could witness and document the evidence: While overactive thyroid was in the stages of development, weight loss was rapid. After treatment, weight returns to normal and stabilizes. Traditionally, the thyroid gland has been thought of as the "weight loss gland," controlling the way that pounds are put on and taken off. This thinking has led to the mistaken notion that giving thyroid medication unnecessarily can promote weight loss. Sometimes people who were taking thyroid hormone supplement did lose significant amounts of weight, adding anecdotal "proof" to support the assumption that the thyroid gland controlled body weight. The thyroid gland became known as the master control for the body's metabolism. There are some kernels of truth here. Certainly weight management is involved with metabolism, which is a function of thyroid activity. But it is also a function of many other factors, both internal and external. In fact, weight management is a good example of the complex nature of our metabolic matrix. First, remember that we are all individuals with different genetic expressions. Some of us can spend all the time we want at the dessert counter without gaining an ounce, while others can walk by a bakery and gain weight. If it were just a matter of proper thyroid function, weight loss in people with normal thyroids would simply be a matter of counting calories, and dieting wouldn't be the frustrating endeavor and billion-dollar industry it is.

We now know that, in addition to thyroid effects, the adrenal gland is intimately involved. Stress increases adrenal hormones like cortisol, thereby making it harder for the body to access its fat stores. Female hormones estrogen and progesterone are involved in both weight gain and weight deposition, so that a woman's body stores fat in different places, places that are more difficult to lose pounds from. (As many women know, a man on the exact same diet as a woman will generally lose weight faster and in greater amounts). To make it more complex, fat cells themselves produce some estrogen. The brain is involved, particularly the craving centers of the hypothalamus. Even the pineal gland, which establishes the rhythmic nature of hormones, seems to affect weight management. There is evidence that the same meal, eaten later in the day, will cause greater gain weight than if eaten earlier.

Other factors are also involved in weight management. Regular exercise promotes the production of certain enzymes like lipoprotein lipase, that helps to break down fats at the cellular level. Fat cells store toxins as most toxins are fat-soluble. Therefore, as weight loss occurs, these toxins are released, leading to the "toxic" feeling that can occur early in weight loss, a feeling that can prevent you from continuing to lose weight. Multiple nutrients like chromium, vitamins E and C, folic acid, and alpha lipoic acid are necessary for good weight management. And of course, there are the influences of diet and heredity.

As complex as it appears to be, a program of weight management is the most significant health challenge facing Americans today, whether or not thyroid imbalance is part of the picture. The health problems related to obesity now outpace the health problems attributed to cigarette smoking. Two-thirds of Americans are overweight, which means they weigh 20 percent more than is healthy for their height. Nearly half of them (one-third of the American population) are obese—they weigh 30 percent more than is healthy.

THYROID IMBALANCE AND YOUR WEIGHT

The correlation between thyroid function and body weight is real, of course, but it's more of a one-way street than you might think (or wish to be the case). When your thyroid is underactive, your metabolism slows—this you already know, because this is one of the key symptoms of hypothyroidism. Not only does your metabolism slow, however, but also it becomes less efficient. So your body needs even less fuel to function. Compounding the situation is that your energy is low, so you don't feel like doing anything. Your activity level drops off, *further lowering* your metabolic efficiency. Sound like a vicious cycle? For many people with underactive thyroid, it is.

If your thyroid is overactive, you might also find yourself struggling to balance your weight. The typical problem with hyperthyroidism is rapid weight loss even in the face of increased appetite and eating. It's not uncommon, surprisingly, for overactive thyroid to result in weight *gain*. Again, you can blame all of those intricate interrelationships that keep your body in a state of equilibrium. Those overabundant thyroid hormones might be causing your body to run at warp speed, but they aren't giving you any more energy. For a while your endocrine matrix can partially compensate by boosting insulin production, which in turn accelerates glucose use and energy production (the companion side of metabolism). But it's a short-lived burst; your endocrine matrix will only allow such compensation to a certain level. So it doesn't take long for you to "burn out," in a sense, and exhaust your energy stores. As well, insulin "locks" fat into the cells, making weight loss more difficult.

With difficulty sleeping to compound the situation, you begin to feel tired all the time—even in spite of feeling "wired" and anxious as a result of the elevated thyroid hormone levels in your blood—and lack the energy to engage in physical activities. And when your activity level drops off, so does your metabolism. If you still have an increased appetite, you're going to be taking in more energy than your body can use. So it's going to store it as—you guessed it—body fat. Weight gain with overactive thyroid is especially common when the cause of your hyperthyroidism is taking too much thyroid hormone supplement to treat hypothyroidism.

Does it make sense, then, to create an artificial environment of overactive thyroid so that you can lose weight? Although there are some alternative practitioners out there who say yes, the real answer is more complex. As we have seen in previous chapters, the proper conversion of T4 to T3 can be influenced in a variety of ways, including the judicious use of T3 itself. However, giving thyroid hormone solely to induce weight loss is NEVER indicated. The health risks of overactive thyroid are simply too high, and there is as yet insufficient evidence that taking thyroid hormones actually results in weight loss—or at least, weight loss without metabolic dysfunction. In fact, as we just discussed, sometimes the opposite happens, and people taking thyroid hormone supplement gain weight, even when they become hyperthyroid.

What about those dietary supplements that proclaim rapid weight loss through "thyroid stimulation" and increased metabolism? Some of these products contain small amounts of desiccated thyroid extract. Others contain iodine-rich kelp and other kinds of seaweed as fillers. Still others contain herbs like ma huang or ephedra, caffeine, and guarana that are called "thermogenic" for their purported ability to increase metabolism. These products can definitely alter your thyroid balance, affecting your metabolism and body weight. (More on this later in this chapter.) But again, this is weight loss (if it occurs) at the high price of metabolic dysfunction and its related health consequences. More often, any weight loss that happens is the result of the reduced intake of food and increased exercise that the product's directions for use also encourage—a much healthier process. To be successful, any natural weight management program needs to affect the entire metabolic matrix, not just one component like thyroid function or even diet.

ASSESSING THE HEALTH SIGNIFICANCE OF YOUR WEIGHT: BODY MASS INDEX (BMI)

Getting your thyroid function back in balance is unquestionably the first and most important step when it comes to getting your weight in balance. After you accomplish that, you need to know just how your weight is affecting your health. For decades, health-care professionals used height-weight charts to determine what was underweight, normal weight, and overweight. By triangulating the point at which your height, weight, and frame size intersected, you or your doctor could identify into which category you fit.

This was all very fine, except for one detail: the categories had nothing to do with anything. They didn't tell you anything about whether your weight was affecting your health, or even whether you weighed what you should. What they told you was simply where you placed in a mass of averages. The height-weight tables that were a staple in doctors' offices for so long actually represented the averages as drawn from mortality statistics! The tables represented an accumulation of information gathered by measuring and weighing people at death. Insurance companies used these actuarial tables, as they were called, to evaluate risk when issuing life insurance policies. It was the earliest recognition that people who were overweight tended to die younger than did people who were of "average" weight. But it wasn't information that anyone used to help people make changes that could help them live longer.

As research began to accumulate in the 1980s and 1990s that linked body weight with specific health conditions, health experts started looking at ways to help people understand what health risks, if any, their weight poses. They came up with a formula called body mass index, or BMI. It organizes categories by height and weight, as did the old tables. But it organizes them according to their correlation to specific health risks, based on statistical data collected from multiple sources and over several decades. For the first time, health-care professionals could substantiate what they'd long suspected: body weight affects health, and the more overweight you are, the more adverse health consequences there are. In 1998, the Heart, Lung, and Blood Institute of the U.S. National Institutes of Health formalized its recommendations for correlating health risk and BMI.

The easiest way to determine your BMI is to:

- Weigh yourself (no clothing)
- Measure your height
- Locate the intersection between your height and weight on the BMI chart
- Identify the two-digit number that is your BMI

For example, if you are 5' 10" and weigh 160 pounds, your BMI is 23. BMI applies to all adults, men and women. BMI does not present an accurate assessment of any health risk associated

Body Mass Index (BMI)

Weight in Pounds

Shaded Areas Show Healthy BMI

Height	100	105	110	115	120	125	130	135	140	145	150	155	160	165	170	175	180	185	190	195	200	205	210
5'1"	18	19	20	21	22	23	24	25	26	27	28	29	30	31	32	33	34	35	36	36	37	38	39
5'2"	18	19	20	21	22	23	24	25	26	26	27	28	29	30	31	32	33	34	35	36	36	37	38
5'3"	17	18	19	20	21	22	23	24	25	26	27	27	28	29	30	31	32	33	34	34	35	36	37
5'4"	17	18	19	20	21	21	22	23	24	25	26	27	28	28	29	30	31	32	33	34	34	35	36
5'5"	16	17	18	19	20	21	22	23	23	24	25	26	27	28	28	29	30	31	32	33	33	34	35
5'6"	16	17	18	19	19	20	21	22	23	24	25	25	26	27	28	29	29	30	31	32	32	33	34
5'7"	15	16	17	18	19	20	20	21	22	23	24	24	25	26	27	27	28	29	30	30	31	32	33
5'8"	15	16	17	18	18	19	20	21	21	22	23	24	25	25	26	27	28	28	29	30	30	31	32
5'9"	14	15	16	17	18	18	19	20	21	21	22	23	24	24	25	26	27	27	28	29	29	30	31
5'10"	14	15	16	17	17	18	19	19	20	21	22	22	23	24	25	25	26	27	28	28	29	29	30
5'11"	14	15	16	16	17	17	18	19	20	20	21	22	22	23	24	25	25	26	27	27	28	29	29
6'0"	13	14	15	16	16	17	18	18	19	20	20	21	22	22	23	24	24	25	26	26	27	28	28
6'1"	13	14	15	15	16	17	17	18	19	19	20	21	21	22	22	23	24	24	25	26	26	27	27
6'2"	12	13	14	15	15	16	17	17	18	19	19	20	21	21	22	23	23	24	24	25	26	26	27
6'3"	12	13	14	14	15	16	16	17	18	18	19	20	20	21	21	22	23	23	24	24	25	26	26
6'4"	12	13	13	14	14	15	16	16	17	18	18	19	20	20	21	21	22	23	23	24	25	25	26

Adapted from: *Clinical Guidelines on the Identification, Evaluation, and Treatment of Overweight and Obesity in Adults.* NHLBI Obesity Education Initiative. National Institutes of Health, 1998.

with your weight if you have a serious illness, are pregnant, or are an intense athlete with high muscle mass (such as a bodybuilder).

Here's how your BMI correlates to your body weight and resulting health risk:

BMI Correlation to Body Weight and Health Risk		
BMI	**Weight**	**Health Risk**
18 or under	Underweight	Metabolic disorders, low blood pressure, slow heart rate
18–25	Healthy	None
25–29	Overweight	Diabetes, high blood pressure, and high blood cholesterol
29 and over	Obese	Diabetes, high blood pressure, high blood cholesterol, certain cancers, coronary artery disease, infertility, osteoarthritis, early death

The higher your BMI, the greater your health risks. Lowering your BMI—losing weight—lowers your health risk. Many health problems related to weight also decrease. It's possible to lower blood pressure and blood cholesterol to the point at which you no longer need to take medication, for example, as your weight and BMI drop.

COULD BEING OVERWEIGHT CAUSE
THYROID IMBALANCE?

At this time the only link between body weight and thyroid imbalance is that thyroid imbalance creates symptoms related to weight. However, there are intriguing connections between body weight and some endocrine imbalances that raise curiosity about similar connections with thyroid function. The most extensively studied connection is that affecting type 2 diabetes. More than 90 percent of people with type 2 diabetes are overweight, and about 60 percent of them are obese (extremely overweight). Over the years, researchers have explored this connection, trying to establish whether diabetes causes overweight or overweight causes diabetes. The evidence supporting the latter—overweight causes, or at least contributes to diabetes—is overwhelming.

Although high blood sugar is a key sign of diabetes, it is not the cause of the condition, as many people commonly believe. Recent research shows that diabetes is a disorder of insulin. Type 1 diabetes, which requires insulin injections, is an autoimmune condition in which the body's immune system turns on the pancreas and destroys the cells that manufacture insulin. Type 2 diabetes, we now know, involves the way cells receive and use insulin—insulin sensitivity, or more accurately, insulin insensitivity.

In type 2 diabetes, the cells become increasingly resistant to insulin. The mechanism that permits insulin molecules to bind with insulin receptors in the cells seems to malfunction. Since insulin is like the "key" that opens the cells to receive glucose, less binding means less glucose in the cells and more glucose circulating in the blood. As diabetes continues to develop, the situation can shift and the opposite situation arises: the cells allow too much insulin to enter, increasing their acceptance of glucose. This increases the amount of energy they burn, which is what sets up the rapid weight loss that is a hallmark sign of the onset of diabetes. The medications that treat type 2 diabetes work by restoring balance to the body's insulin sensitivity balance.

Recently new understanding has developed about why insulin becomes elevated and insulin resistance occurs. Insulin response to glucose in the body and certain foods are most responsible for rapid increases in blood glucose. Those foods are carbohydrates, particularly grain-based carbohydrates and potatoes. Even sugar needs to be altered a bit before it becomes pure glucose, but grains generally and white flour particularly are pure glucose molecules strung together. All foods can be rated by their "glycemic index," which measures how fast the food can convert into glucose. Refined grains and white potatoes have the highest glycemic index, raise blood glucose the fastest, and therefore stimulate insulin the most.

Twenty-five percent of people are even more sensitive to carbohydrates and their effects on insulin. The results of the chronically elevated insulin levels include more than just weight gain and type 2 diabetes. These people develop higher levels of hypertension, elevated cholesterol, and arteriosclerosis, and even a condition in females called polycystic ovaries. Together, this disarrangement of the metabolic matrix is known as Syndrome X, or the metabolic syndrome. The easiest way to recognize whether you might be in this 25 percent that is at risk for Syndrome X is the waist-to-hip ratio. People with carbohydrate sensitivity are "apple" shaped; that is, they have weight in their waist, with thinner limbs and hips. People with less of this problem are more "pear" shaped, meaning their hips are larger than their waist size. A simple measurement can, therefore, give a hint as to the healthiest diet for you.

Its treatment, simply enough, is to limit grain-based carbohydrates (vegetable carbohydrates generally have a lower glycemic index). While this dietary change flies in the face of decades of warnings to lose weight by "cutting out fat," it should be obvious that (for some people at least), this approach does not work. Studies show that the U.S. diet has decreased in fat over the past two decades (largely due to the low-fat movement), but obesity and cholesterol have increased.

Researchers believe that excess body fat contributes to diabetes, rather than the other way around, because they can create diabetes in test animals in controlled laboratory settings just by creating obesity in the animals. There is increasing evidence that when body fat reaches a certain point—extreme obesity—insulin imbalance is certain. When body weight decreases, insulin balance shifts back toward normal. Of course, people who have healthy body weight also develop diabetes, so clearly there are multiple factors involved in the condition. Overweight is a significant contributing factor in diabetes, but not the sole cause.

This correlation raises interest in whether it also exists in other endocrine-based conditions, such as thyroid and adrenal imbalance, because changes in body weight are often among the symptoms. It's particularly intriguing when looking at thyroid balance, as thyroid hormone and insulin are instrumental elements of the two components of metabolism. What seems to make this correlation different is that although type 2 diabetes typically improves with weight loss, thyroid function does not. Current treatment focuses on restoring the balance of thyroid hormone in the body. But as our understanding of the body's intricate interrelationships grows and deepens, we're looking more intently at these kinds of correlations.

UNDERWEIGHT AND HEALTH PROBLEMS

Being underweight carries its own set of risks related to health. These can be just as serious as the health risks related to being overweight. But our "thin is in" culture tends to overlook this reality. When your body weight drops below 95 percent of what is a healthy weight for you according to your BMI, your risks for health problems take a significant jump. Signs that body weight is too low can include sensitivity to cold and heat, low blood pressure, and slow heart rate.

Sometimes metabolic disorders develop, such as diabetes insipidus (a disorder affecting the pituitary gland, not the same condition we commonly think of as diabetes). Other signs of metabolic changes can include a yellow tint to the skin, reflecting the body's growing inability to metabolize beta carotene into vitamin A. And underweight affects both insulin sensitivity and thyroid function, further altering your body's metabolic functions and balance.

In Chapter 3 we talked about the role of the thyroid gland as your body's metabolic thermostat. Part of its function is to keep your body alive when it's facing starvation. When your body fat drops below a certain level (usually when your weight is 90 percent lower than is healthy), your endocrine matrix interprets this as impending starvation. It begins to issue hormonal directives:

- Your adrenal glands lower production of hormones such as cortisol and adrenaline, helping to lower your heart rate and slow your breathing.
- Your thyroid gland decreases hormone production, and T4-to-T3 conversion slows to limit thyroid hormone availability to your cells.
- Cell function slows due to lack of thyroid hormone to fuel the ATP production of the cells.
- Your pancreas cuts back on insulin production because your cells are burning less energy and so need less glucose.
- Your body temperature lowers, further lowering energy needs.

You don't realize it, but your body has essentially prepared itself for a state of near-hibernation. Your body is not receiving the nutrients it needs, so it is shutting down nonessential functions to be sure that vital organs like your brain and your heart continue to receive enough fuel to keep you alive.

The health risks of being underweight can be particularly serious if an eating disorder is the reason for the weight imbalance. Anorexia nervosa, in which the sufferer eats too little to sustain the functions of the body in a healthy state, can cause sudden cardiac death even in someone who is young. Bulimia and bingeing, which can involve forced vomiting and/or diuretic use, can cause damage to the esophagus, mouth, and teeth. Untreated, eating disorders keep the body in a constant state of near-starvation, and body functions begin to shut down to ensure the body's survival. This includes changes in insulin sensitivity and in thyroid function, both of which affect metabolism.

Underweight is also associated with fertility problems, especially in women. A woman's body composition includes more fat, by percentage, than a man's body to accommodate a woman's role in bearing children. Body fat represents stored energy that the woman's body can call on if needed. Fat cells also make small amounts of estrogen, one of the hormones necessary for sustaining pregnancy and for breastfeeding. (See Chapter 18 for more about fertility and thyroid.)

Just as underactive thyroid is not solely responsible for being overweight, overactive thyroid is only partially responsible for being underweight. The majority of people with hyperthyroidism might lose 10 to 20 pounds and then plateau; fewer than 10 percent actually continue to lose weight as a result of thyroid imbalance. As well, most people with overactive thyroid regain lost weight once treatment succeeds in correcting the thyroid imbalance.

DO YOU WEIGH TOO MUCH,
TOO LITTLE, OR JUST RIGHT?

Three in four people underestimate their weight and the amount of food they eat, or overestimate the level of physical activity in their lives. Are you among them? Your answers to these questions might provide surprising information about how your lifestyle influences both your body weight and your health. Check the response that best applies to you.

LIFESTYLE QUIZ

1. At meal times, I eat . . .
   - ☐ Until there are no more servings available.
   - ☐ Large portions of the foods I like and no foods I don't like.
   - ☐ Small portions of different kinds of foods.
   - ☐ Until I'm full.

2. In the course of a day, I snack on . . .
   - ☐ Chips and snack crackers.
   - ☐ Cookies, pastries, and candy.
   - ☐ Fresh fruits and vegetables.
   - ☐ Nothing; I don't snack.

3. I shop primarily . . .
   - ☐ At the local convenience store.
   - ☐ In the middle aisles of the supermarket.
   - ☐ Around the perimeter of the supermarket.
   - ☐ From vending machines.

4. A slice of bread is . . .
   - ☐ A means of getting other foods into our mouths.
   - ☐ To be accompanied by a jug of wine and thou.

☐ An easy way to raise insulin levels.
☐ One of the main ingredients of toast.

5. The physical activity I get each day is usually . . .
   ☐ Walking to and from my car.
   ☐ Parking my car at least the distance of a block from my destination and walking the rest of the way.
   ☐ Taking the stairs instead of the elevator.
   ☐ Walking or bicycling to work.

6. The physical activity I get in the course of a week is usually . . .
   ☐ Grocery shopping, housework, and cleaning.
   ☐ Playing with the kids.
   ☐ Brisk walking for 30 minutes, three or four days a week.
   ☐ Planned exercise and fitness activities three or four days a week.

7. The distance I can walk without getting winded is about . . .
   ☐ From my car to the door.
   ☐ Down three flights of stairs.
   ☐ Around the block.
   ☐ Up three flights of stairs.

8. Physical difficulties that keep me from being active include . . .
   ☐ Easily tire or get winded.
   ☐ Joints ache.
   ☐ No one to do things with me.
   ☐ Don't have the gear or clothing for the activities that interest me.

There aren't right or wrong answers to these questions; they are only to help you identify some of your current lifestyle habits. Here's what your responses might suggest:

1. Ours is a "supersize" culture. We equate more with better. And if we can get more *faster*, even better! But what we consider to be a "portion" or serving size is often two to six times larger than what it actually is. A serving size of soda, for example, is 6 ounces. Yet a can of soda is 12 ounces, and a fast-food restaurant soda might be 16, 28, or 32 ounces. We also tend to support the "clean plate club"—if it's on your plate, you eat it because to leave it is to be wasteful. But when it comes to eating habits, what this really means is more body weight, faster. Two-thirds of Americans weigh more than is healthy, and the volume of food we consume is a main reason. Some of the more successful weight management programs, such as Weight Watchers, focus largely on portion control.

2. Most people snack during the day. We get hungry or thirsty; we have something to eat or drink. In and of itself, this is not a bad thing. In fact, nutritionists believe we would all have healthier eating habits if we ate five or six small meals spread throughout the day. Unfortunately, the snack foods that are most convenient are also the most nutritionally empty—chips, crackers, cookies, candy, soda. They add calories but little else. Furthermore, they have a high glycemic index, raising insulin levels. Fresh fruits and vegetables have nutritional value and help you feel full longer.

3. One thing unites the corner grocery store, the mega-supermarket, and even the natural foods stores: the protein, fresh fruits, and vegetables are strewn around the outside of the store, while row after row of flour products

and other carbohydrates fill the inside of the store. A good rule of thumb is to do two-thirds of your shopping in the outer portion of the supermarket. We call this diet the protein-and-produce diet. The remaining one-third should focus on whole-grain carbohydrates, which have lower glycemic indices than refined carbohydrates.

The past few decades have taken their dietary leadership from the U.S. Department of Agriculture's Food Pyramid, which put grains at the wide bottom. This certainly was an improvement over the previous fat-laden meat-and-potatoes U.S. diet. But we now are beginning to realize that the food pyramid is outmoded, that the refined carbohydrates that dominate fast food and American diets generally can lead to dangerously high insulin levels and a variety of diseases and medical conditions.

So, our recommendations are to limit the breads, crackers, chips, donuts, pastas, rice, sweetened fast foods, and soft drinks in the diet. We stress the importance of whole-grain breads and grains when they are eaten.

And, we suggest following a protein-and-produce diet. This means choosing a salad with strips of chicken or shrimp rather than a sandwich for lunch, fruit and nuts with unsweetened yogurt or a whole-grain cereal for breakfast, and a moderate portion of baked or broiled protein, with salad and vegetables for dinner. Snacks can be nuts and fruit, yogurt, cheese, or a protein shake or bar. Restaurant choices can include a chicken cutlet, nonbreaded, with vegetables and salad at an Italian restaurant, leaving the bread and pasta. A glass of red wine, with its strong antioxidant content, tops off the meal. When dining in a Chinese restaurant, stir-fry chicken or fish and vegetables, leaving the rice aside, make good choices. Even fast-food places are catering to salad-craving customers. A salad accompanied by a protein source, with the breading removed, makes a good choice in a pinch. And always, leave the sweet-ened desserts for special occasions.

4. Fewer than one in ten Americans get enough physical activity in their daily lives. In this era of electronic gad-getry and extended commuting, more people have lifestyles in which they need to walk only from their cars to their desks, and from their cars to their couches. We instead must make time for, and put effort into, physical activity. Regular physical activity improves the efficiency of cell functions, allowing cells to make better use of nutrients and hormones such as thyroid hormone and insulin.

5. Regular exercise—physical activity that increases heart rate—improves heart health. Health experts recom-mend a minimum of 30 minutes of physical activity, such as walking, three to four days a week, and 60 min-utes of more strenuous exercise three to four days a week. However, even more moderate exercise can aid in weight loss by encouraging your body to produce the enzymes that break down fat.

6. There are a number of elaborate formulas for figuring out your fitness level. But one very simple approach is to determine how far you can walk before getting winded. If you can walk up three flights of stairs without huffing and puffing, your fitness level is prob-ably good. If you have trouble breathing without panting after walking from your door to your car, or can't walk around the block without stopping to catch your breath, your fitness level is unhealthy.

7. Being overweight interferes with physical activity in a number of ways. Fortunately, most of them go away as you lose weight. Carrying around 20 percent more weight (or more) than you should puts a considerable

burden on body systems not really designed to handle such a load. It affects your flexibility and strength. It puts added pressure on weight-bearing joints such as your hips, knees, and ankles. Motivation is also a factor. It's more fun to walk or exercise with others. Many people find enrolling in programs through fitness clubs or gyms gives physical activity a more social context and increases their motivation to regularly participate.

HOW TO LOSE WEIGHT

The best way to lose weight is to first restore your thyroid balance. Both underactive and overactive thyroid can leave you feeling lethargic and disinterested—you have little interest in anything except resting or sleeping. This is because thyroid imbalance throws your metabolism out of kilter. Not only do you feel that you have no energy; you actually don't. Your cells are not able to make ATP, your body's long-term energy supply, without adequate thyroid hormone. And even if you have too much thyroid hormone, as with hyperthyroidism, the increased metabolic rate that results burns the ATP in an effort to keep up with your body's intensified demands for energy. The only way to interrupt this cycle is to restore balance to your thyroid.

The next step is to change the habits that have caused you to gain weight. Dieting—eating in a special way for a certain amount of time—seldom achieves lasting results. In fact, 80 percent of people who diet gain back lost pounds and more within three years. The main reason that diets fail is that they are temporary. A diet is oriented toward meeting a specific and narrowly defined goal, such as to lose 20 pounds. Once the goal is met, the effort expended toward meeting it stops. You're back to your old ways . . . and before you know it, you're back to your old weight, too.

Rather than helping you to change your eating habits over the long term, most diets require severe restrictions that are impossible and unhealthy to sustain. Your ultimate goal is not just to lose weight but also to keep it off so that you can maintain a healthy balance. This requires changing your perspectives about food and the *way* you eat, not just *what* you eat. In general, your weight loss efforts are more likely to succeed when you:

- Lose weight gradually, no faster than one-half to one pound a week (four to five pounds a month). Weight loss that is faster than this is very likely to trigger your body's starvation response, which lowers your metabolism to preserve your energy resources.
- Lose no more than 20 percent of your body weight over the course of a year. This means that if your weight is significantly more than is healthy, it might take you several years to bring it down to a healthy point. But it's far more likely that you'll be able to keep it there.
- Cut down on grains and sweetened foods generally, and refined carbohydrates specifically. Shop around the perimeter of your supermarket. Follow the protein-and-produce diet, with some whole grains added.
- Eat the foods you like, in moderation. Take small portions, and ask yourself whether you're truly still hungry or just want more of the food when you reach for additional servings. (If you're not sure about portion sizes, try this: take what you would usually take, and then put half of it back.)
- Eat when you are hungry rather than at defined times, and eat only as much food as it takes for you to feel full. At first it might seem a nuisance, but it helps you tune in to your body's needs. More often than not, we eat at mealtimes because we've programmed ourselves to eat when the clock tells us it's time.

- Increase your physical activity. Walk as much as possible. If you find it hard to walk for 30 minutes at a time, walk for 15 minutes at a time, twice a day. Do this every day to make it a pattern of daily life. Regular physical activity also helps you to build muscle mass, and muscle tissues burn more calories than fat tissues.
- Exercise. This pushes your body to develop greater efficiency. Choose moderately strenuous activities that you enjoy: jogging, swimming, bicycling, roller-skating, tennis, basketball. Choose some activities that you can do by yourself, and others that you can do with a partner or a group.

HOW TO GAIN WEIGHT

If your thyroid is overactive, you might struggle to keep your body weight high enough. Generally, once your thyroid hormone balance returns to normal this is no longer a problem from a metabolic perspective. To gain weight in a healthy way:

- Plan regular meals, and eat them as planned. Make sure to eat plenty of good quality protein, especially if you are exercising regularly.
- Plan nutritious snacks. This assures that your body has a steady supply of nutrients throughout the day, offsetting peaks and valleys in your metabolism.
- Get regular physical activity to help your body run at peak efficiency. Staying active also increases your appetite, encouraging you to eat more.
- Weight training is not just for body builders. Even light weight training is helpful to prevent osteoporosis and to control the symptoms of arthritis. A weight program will help to build muscle and increase weight in a proper manner.

If your weight fails to return to a healthy point (BMI between 18 and 25), there could be other factors at play. It would be a good idea to have a thorough physical exam, and discuss with your doctor the ways in which your weight may be affecting your health.

FINDING YOUR HEALTHY WEIGHT

There is no such thing as a "perfect" weight. You are an individual, with unique needs. The weight that is right for you might not be right for someone else of similar stature. What is most important is that your body weight supports your good health rather than stands in the way of it.

17

Managing Your Thyroid with Other Serious Health Problems

Having a thyroid imbalance and other health conditions can affect treatment for both your thyroid and the other conditions. Sometimes the drugs you're taking for treatment interact with each other, while at other times the conditions themselves generate interactions that need monitoring or managing. Taking good care of your health—all of your health—means balancing the sometimes differing needs of these conditions.

THYROID BALANCE AND OTHER ENDOCRINE CONDITIONS

Thyroid balance goes hand-in-hand with balance all along your endocrine matrix. When one component is out of kilter, the others attempt to compensate. Sometimes this is successful, at least in the short term, and sometimes it creates additional problems. Prolonged, untreated underactive thyroid, for example, stresses the adrenal glands. This can result in adrenal fatigue.

Doctors diagnose endocrine disorders by looking at the combination of your symptoms and the test results that measure relevant hormones in your body. Some endocrine disorders, like diabetes, are clear. Others, like adrenal fatigue, take some detective work to unravel.

Treating one endocrine disorder affects function and balance across the endocrine matrix, too. When treatment restores thyroid balance, the stress the thyroid has been putting on the adrenal glands eases. The adrenals can then back off on their efforts (although they sometimes need a therapeutic boost to help their function return to normal). Chapters 2 and 4 discuss the intricate interrelationships of the endocrine matrix, both in health and in dysfunction.

THYROID BALANCE AND OTHER AUTOIMMUNE CONDITIONS

Autoimmune response causes about 90 percent of thyroid imbalance, both underactive and overactive. The autoimmune disorder Graves' disease is the most common form of hyperthyroidism; its counterpart on the hypothyroid side is Hashimoto's thyroiditis. Both conditions involve your immune system, producing antibodies that attack your thyroid tissue. If you have one autoimmune disorder, you're at increased risk for others. (Chapter 9 discusses the body's immune and autoimmune responses.)

Some of the symptoms of hyperthyroidism are separate autoimmune responses themselves. Infiltrative ophthalmopathy (involving the eyes) and infiltrative dermopathy (involving the skin) are conditions that develop in conjunction with overactive thyroid, but then run their own courses. Treating the hyperthyroidism may or may not influence their symptoms and progression. These conditions do not develop without the presence of hyperthyroidism, although they can show up years before or after the hyperthyroidism.

If you have thyroid imbalance, either underactive or overactive, consider this a "heads up" for remaining vigilant about symptoms that you might develop that suggest other autoimmune conditions. Early intervention and treatment if necessary often make the difference between a condition you can manage and a condition that starts to manage you. Some of the common autoimmune disorders that are often present or develop when you have autoimmune thyroid include:

Common Autoimmune Disorders Associated with Autoimmune Thyroid		
Condition	**Body System Affected**	**Symptoms**
Ankylosing spondylitis	Spine	Pain that begins in lower back and spreads upward along the spine
Diabetes	Pancreas (endocrine)	Rapid weight loss, lack of energy
Myasthenia gravis	Muscles	Muscle weakness and difficulty moving
Pernicious anemia	Stomach lining	Weakness; sore tongue and bleeding gums; tingling in legs and arms
Polyglandular deficiency syndrome	Multiple endocrine glands	Vary according to the glands that are involved
Rheumatoid arthritis	Joints and cartilage	Joint pain and swelling; general tiredness; low-grade fever; weight loss
Scleroderma	Connective tissue	Pain and tenderness of skin surface and joints; tight, shiny-looking skin
Systemic lupus erythematosus	Random	Fever and chills; fatigue; weight loss; "butterfly" rash on the face; irregular periods in women

Other conditions known to have autoimmune components include ulcerative colitis, psoriasis, and multiple sclerosis. Autoimmune conditions can be difficult to diagnose, and tend to run in families. Check your family medical history to find out whether any autoimmune conditions exist among your relatives. It doesn't have to be the same condition, like diabetes, to establish a connection, just anything autoimmune. Keep this information handy, so that if you do develop symptoms, you can share your family medical history with your doctor. And remember: knowledge is power. Knowing what to look for doesn't "create" the presence of the disorder. Instead, it gives you the edge in minimizing the effects that autoimmune conditions can have on your life and your lifestyle.

Like most illnesses, autoimmune problems are a complex interplay of genetics and environmental factors, both internal and external. Diet, pollution, stress, infection, and even medically administered treatments such as antibiotics and vaccines have been implicated as having roles in the development of autoimmunity. The digestive tract is lined with antibodies, and many natural treatments for autoimmune conditions, including thyroid imbalance, focus on the health of the gut.

THYROID BALANCE AND HEART DISEASE

Although Chapter 14 discusses in detail the relationship between heart disease and thyroid imbalance, it's worth mentioning a few key points here. First, *untreated* thyroid disorders inevitably lead to the conditions of heart disease. Untreated hyperthyroidism is a faster path to heart problems, but untreated hypothyroidism eventually catches up. The nature of your thyroid imbalance—underactive or overactive—determines the specific components of heart disease that develop, but the end result is still a significant risk to your heart and to your life.

Once hyperthyroidism is under control through treatment,

it no longer poses a threat to your heart health. That's not quite the case with hypothyroidism. Dangerous increases in blood cholesterol levels and homocysteine levels (another diet-based substance that contributes to arterial disease) do decline with treatment for underactive thyroid, which lowers one risk factor. But in a somewhat unfair fashion, untreated hypothyroidism actually *helps* a heart condition called ischemic heart disease. (But not enough to justify the other risks of allowing underactive thyroid to remain untreated.)

Ischemia is a condition in which tissues don't receive enough oxygen, almost always because the arteries that supply them with blood are narrowed or blocked. When oxygen demand exceeds supply in the affected tissues, they sound the alarm through pain signals. You ease what you're doing, the oxygen demand drops, and the pain stops. Ischemia can affect just about any tissue—kidneys, brain, legs. When it affects your heart, then it's caused by coronary artery disease and is called ischemic heart disease.

By slowing the metabolism of heart cells just as it slows the metabolism of cells throughout your body, hypothyroidism reduces their need for oxygen. This, of course, reduces their demand for oxygen, and makes it seem as though everything is fine with your heart. If your ischemic heart disease is undiagnosed and your doctor starts you on thyroid hormone supplement, there's a rude awakening just around the corner. As your metabolism returns to normal, those heart cells wake up. They need and want more oxygen to fuel their activities. When they don't get it, you feel the pain—called angina when it comes from your heart. If the degree of ischemic heart disease is moderate to significant, the restoration of normal metabolism could be enough to send you into a heart attack.

If you are over age 50 or have a family history of heart disease, have your doctor check you for ischemic heart disease before prescribing thyroid hormone supplement for you. There are a number of ways your doctor can test for the presence of coronary artery disease. If you know you have coronary artery disease, or if you have angina, then your doctor will probably start you out on fairly low doses of thyroid hormone supplement and slowly work you up to a level that relieves your thyroid imbalance without exacerbating your heart problems. And of course, you'll want to follow up with your doctor for appropriate treatment to restore your heart to health.

THYROID BALANCE, CHRONIC FATIGUE SYNDROME, AND FIBROMYALGIA

Chronic fatigue syndrome (CFS) is a collection of symptoms clustered around the core symptom of fatigue. There are no tests to specifically determine that CFS exists. Rather, it is a process of diagnosis by elimination. After all other potential causes of the symptoms have been dismissed, the last diagnosis remaining is chronic fatigue syndrome. This process is frustrating for patients and doctors alike. There are dozens of symptoms that are linked to CFS. Not everyone who has the disease has all of the symptoms, and symptoms tend to occur in different groupings or patterns in the people who have them. In short, there is very little that is consistent or predictable about CFS.

Fibromyalgia has symptoms similar to those of CFS, but they cluster around the core symptom of moderate to severe pain in the joints. Like CFS, fibromyalgia is at the end of the diagnostic chain, reached when all other diagnoses are ruled out. As well, most people with fibromyalgia have "tender point" sensitivity that helps narrow the diagnostic range. Some doctors believe that fibromyalgia is a complication or progression of CFS, while others believe it is an independent autoimmune disorder similar to but not related to rheumatoid arthritis.

Treatment for these conditions targets relieving their symptoms, and generally encompasses a wide range of therapies from drugs (such as NSAIDs, steroids, antidepressants) to meditation, biofeedback, yoga, acupuncture, and nutritional therapy. In the mid-1990s researchers for the first time detected a link to low T3 levels in people who have these conditions. Some researchers speculate that underactive thyroid is at the root of the diverse and numerous symptoms, and that as an autoimmune disorder itself hypothyroidism initiates a sequence of events that subsequently launches other autoimmune attacks.

If you have thyroid imbalance *and* CFS or fibromyalgia, it's important to stay on top of your thyroid function. Have blood thyroid levels tested every six months, at least for the first couple of years after your diagnosis, to make sure your T3 levels are adequate. If you have either CFS or fibromyalgia (or suspect that you do) but haven't been tested for thyroid function, it's time for a trip to the doctor. Not only do more than half of those who have CFS and fibromyalgia have underactive thyroid, but also ongoing research suggests hypothyroidism might be the staging ground for these conditions.

THYROID BALANCE AND CANCER

There are two ways thyroid and cancer can cross paths: when cancer involves the thyroid, and when cancer involves another part of the body. Cancer involving the thyroid gland is relatively rare, and usually easy to treat in that cancerous thyroid tumors are slow to spread. The first stage of treatment is surgery to remove the lobe of the thyroid gland that contains the tumor. If the tumor is large or if there are multiple tumors, it's necessary to remove the entire thyroid gland.

Sometimes the next stage of treatment is radioactive iodine, just to be sure there are no stray cancer cells lingering in remaining thyroid tissue. This treatment is called thyroid ablation. The final stage of treatment for thyroid cancer is to suppress TSH stimulation of thyroid activity by taking thyroid hormone supplement. The intent is to create a permanent state of functional hypothyroidism. This treatment is lifelong, and keeps thyroid tissue from becoming active again. As long as thyroid tissue is nonfunctional, it can't support a recurring tumor.

When there is cancer in another part of the body, your focus shifts to doing what is necessary to contain it—and rightfully so. Problems like thyroid balance seem minor compared to the potential consequences of something as serious as cancer. But today there are many treatments for cancer that produce successful outcomes—they send cancer into remission or cure it completely.

Cancers in other locations affect thyroid function in various ways, just as any imbalance elsewhere in the body affects thyroid balance. Hormone-driven cancers such as breast cancer, uterine cancer (in women), and prostate cancer (in men) alter the endocrine matrix. Treatments that affect hormone balance alter the endocrine matrix, too. And as Chapter 2 discusses, what affects one point on the matrix affects all other points.

Cancer and cancer treatment often affect nutrition. Chemotherapy and radiation therapy can leave you feeling weak and nauseated, and not very interested in eating. This can affect the amounts of iodine and tyrosine, the key ingredients of thyroid hormone, which you provide for your thyroid gland. General nutritional deficiencies affect cell metabolism in ways too numerous to discuss here.

If you also have underactive thyroid and are taking thyroid hormone supplement, the changes in your eating habits as well as the changes in your metabolism will affect how your body absorbs and uses the supplement. And if you are taking nutritional supplements to counteract the effects of cancer or cancer treatment, they could contain substances—even minerals such as calcium and iron—that affect how your body absorbs and uses thyroid supplement.

If you are receiving treatment for cancer, discuss the possible ramifications the treatment might have on your thyroid imbalance and what effects your thyroid condition might have on the cancer as well as its treatment. Sometimes there are interactions between drugs used to treat other symptoms and the thyroid hormone supplement you take to control your thyroid. Your doctor or pharmacist can help you figure out if there are any potential interactions that should concern you, and help you determine how to accommodate them without jeopardizing your health.

Radiation treatment for cancers affecting the lymph nodes in your neck (such as with Hodgkin's disease and non-Hodgkin's lymphoma) or for cancers involving structures of your neck and mouth can also affect your thyroid gland. It's very hard to mask off the thyroid gland to protect it from being irradiated at the same time. Although today's radiation treatments are very narrowly focused and targeted, some exposure to healthy tissues occurs. This can end up poisoning thyroid tissue, resulting in hypothyroidism.

If you are receiving or have received treatment for cancer, it's a good idea to have your blood thyroid levels checked at least every six months, and more frequently if you have symptoms of thyroid imbalance. If you have radiation treatment to your neck, face, or upper chest, have thyroid blood tests done every three months until it appears clear that your thyroid remains healthy.

THYROID BALANCE AND SKIN PROBLEMS

Both underactive and overactive thyroid generate skin problems. Dry, itchy, flaky skin is a hallmark symptom of underactive thyroid. Soft skin, darkened pigmentation, and reddened face sometimes occur with overactive thyroid. Both generally return to normal when your thyroid balance does. One exception is the leathery lesions of infiltrative dermopathy that can occur with Graves' disease (hyperthyroidism). These might fade but generally remain visible.

The skin changes associated with hyperthyroidism usually aren't as prominent or persistent as those linked with hypothyroidism, and go away early in the treatment process. Except for infiltrative dermopathy, which often itches, the skin changes of overactive thyroid don't usually warrant any kind of treatment other than good skin care for general skin health.

The skin changes that occur with hypothyroidism are another story. To care for your skin when you have hypothyroidism, start by drinking lots of water—at least 8 to 12 full glasses every day. An adequate fluid volume is the best possible moisturizer for your skin, and helps keep other body systems healthy, too. Use gentle soap, and shower or bathe in water that is warm but not hot. Soaking in a tub of water is both relaxing and good for your skin—again, in warm but not hot water. After showering or bathing, and frequently throughout the day, apply a moisturizing cream or lotion to your hands, feet, knees, elbows, face, and other areas that you know are prone to dryness.

Underactive thyroid causes changes to your hair, too. You might lose hair in various places on your body. Some people lose circular patches on their heads, a condition called alopecia areata, which is itself an autoimmune condition. You might find that the hair on your head becomes coarse and brittle. It's also common to lose the hair on the outer portions of your eyebrows. Generally, these problems, like skin problems, end when treatment restores your thyroid balance. Lost hair usually but not always returns (although the patches of alopecia areata often remain).

Continued skin problems after your treatment for hypothyroidism (thyroid hormone supplement) is well under way could mean that your supplement dose isn't quite right or that you have skin problems not related to thyroid balance. If your skin problems continue, see a dermatologist (doctor specializing in caring for skin conditions) and also have your regular doctor check your blood thyroid levels.

THYROID BALANCE AND MEDICATIONS FOR COLDS AND ALLERGIES

Read the label on just about any over-the-counter product to relieve the symptoms of colds or allergies. In the "Do not use this product if . . ." listing you'll find ". . . you have thyroid disease." This leads you to think that either taking the product will make your thyroid condition worse or having a thyroid condition means the medication won't work properly for you. Neither is correct.

This warning applies to the decongestant component of the product. Decongestants—pseudoephedrine is the most common one—act as stimulants. They increase your heart rate and respirations, and might make you feel a bit "wired." You can experience the same symptoms with overactive thyroid, or if you have underactive thyroid but are taking more thyroid hormone supplement than you need and it's creating a situation of false or temporary hyperthyroidism. Stimulants can sometimes affect thyroid function, either depressing or accelerating thyroid hormone production.

Although allergy preparations generally contain an antihistamine, which is *not* a stimulant, to block the allergic response in your body, many of them also contain a decongestant to help relieve the stuffiness you might be feeling, especially when you have seasonal allergies (also called hay fever). If the effects of such products generate unpleasant symptoms for you, try using an allergy product that contains just an antihistamine. A drugstore's pharmacist can help you identify these products.

The drawback to using a straight antihistamine is that most of them, at least those that are available without a doctor's prescription, cause drowsiness. One of the most popular, diphenhydramine (as in the brand-name product Benadryl), is so noted for its ability to cause sleepiness that it's also used as the main ingredient in many over-the-counter sleep aids! If you need an antihistamine and also need to stay awake and alert, ask your doctor to write a prescription for one of the newer antihistamine drugs that do not cause drowsiness. You might also try a natural antihistamine such as vitamin C or quercitin. But remember, too much quercitin can itself affect T3 production. Always follow the dosage directions on the product label.

When you have a cold, the decongestant component might be just as important to you as the antihistamine, as that's what relieves stuffiness and congestion, clearing your sinuses so you can move air through them again. Try buying the antihistamine and the decongestant separately, and take just half a dose of the decongestant. This should cause fewer stimulant symptoms, and is likely to give you at least partial relief. To avoid any possibility of creating problems with your thyroid balance, however, consider using natural remedies rather than drugs to relieve sinus and nasal congestion. Some that provide prompt relief with no side effects include:

- Breathe steam. Boil water in a teakettle and breathe in the steam (be careful not to get close enough to burn yourself). Or turn on the hot water in the shower, close the bathroom door, and let the steam fill the room. Turn off the hot water and sit in the bathroom, breathing in the steam.
- Use saline nose drops. You can buy a commercial preparation or mix your own with salt and water. Tilt your head back, and with a dropper place two or three drops in each nostril. Hold your head back for a few minutes to let the mixture penetrate. Have tissues handy!
- Sit in the cool, moist, night air. This is a favorite remedy among parents for children who have croup, a barky

cough caused by congestion that lodges in the throat and upper chest. The cool moisture helps to break up the congestion so you can breathe. And it's relaxing to sit out under the night sky and watch the stars.

- Some herbal decongestants contain ephedra, or ma huang. Although this herb shrinks nasal passages and in fact is the basis for the drug pseudoephedrine, *do not take it* if you have hypertension (high blood pressure), heart disease, or kidney disease. Generally, you should not take ephedra unless under a skilled, licensed health care practitioner's direction.
- Bromelain, an enzyme from pineapple that breaks down protein structures, can help to clear mucous if taken between meals. One study suggested that taking bromelain helped antibiotics to penetrate mucous-laden tissues in sinusitis.
- N-acetyl cysteine, or NAC, is a natural amino acid. In the body, it breaks up mucous and is useful in sinus congestion. In its synthetic form, marketed as the brand-name product Mucomist, this drug is used in hospitals to treat the congestion of asthma.

Some people like to use aromatic lozenges to help relieve nasal congestion. These work by releasing a mild irritant, such as menthol, when you suck on them. The irritant causes your nasal passages to dilate and the secretions to become thin. The resulting drainage then clears blocked breathing passages. Sometimes the irritant ingredient turns out to be more irritating than you're willing to tolerate.

THYROID BALANCE AND YOUR EMOTIONS

The relationship of thyroid and other hormones to mood and cognition is a clear example of the metabolic matrix at work. The neurotransmitters serotonin, dopamine, and norepinephrine function in concert to balance your mood (among other functions). When there is more of one and less of the others, the balance shifts. The functions of your cognitive processes—thinking, memory, concentration—depend on this balance. So do your moods and your emotions. Thyroid hormone affects this balance through its actions within the endocrine matrix and also on the metabolism of brain cells. Brain cells have T3 receptors, making them directly responsive to thyroid hormone.

New medications to treat depression, called serotonin reuptake inhibitors (SSRIs), increase the levels of serotonin in the brain by preventing its breakdown. This improves mood, relieving depression. New research suggests that T3 plays a key role in this process. When T3 levels are low, SSRIs are less effective. When T3 levels rise, serotonin levels rise and SSRIs become more effective at keeping them up. A number of psychiatrists are now adding low-dose T3 therapy to the treatment regimen for depression, which seems to help many people improve faster.

People with other psychiatric conditions related to neurotransmitter imbalances, such as obsessive-compulsive disorder and bipolar disorder, often have underactive thyroid. Although restoring thyroid balance doesn't necessarily end the psychiatric symptoms, the drugs to treat those symptoms work better when thyroid balance is normal. Sometimes people with thyroid imbalance are misdiagnosed with, and treated incorrectly for, psychiatric illnesses. This is most likely to happen when other typical symptoms of thyroid imbalance are not present.

An overactive thyroid can cause dopamine and norepinephrine levels to rise and serotonin levels to drop, resulting in:

- Feelings of tension and anxiety
- Extreme and rapid mood swings, from exhilaration to paranoia and rage (clinically known as emotional lability)
- Irritability and impatience

- Hyperactivity
- Heightened sensitivity to noise
- Inability to sleep

Treating these symptoms without treating the underlying thyroid imbalance seldom succeeds. Restoring thyroid balance often, but not always, ends psychiatric symptoms. Sometimes it is necessary to treat both problems until the symptoms are under control, and then gradually decrease drug doses.

An underactive thyroid can cause serotonin and norepinephrine levels to drop and dopamine levels to rise, resulting in:

- Lack of interest in daily activities
- "Foggy" cognitive functions
- Diminished short-term memory
- Blandness of personality
- Suspicion and paranoia

Treating the underlying thyroid imbalance is again crucial for gaining control over these symptoms. Sometimes depression lingers after thyroid balance returns, requiring continued treatment. Many doctors combine T3 treatment with antidepressant drugs to tackle both imbalances at once. This is typically a more successful strategy than attacking each separately. Regular follow-up is important, so your doctor can adjust your doses as your symptoms change and improve.

Lithium, a drug commonly prescribed to treat bipolar disorder (once called manic-depressive disorder), interferes with the thyroid gland's hormone production processes. It might also interfere with T4-to-T3 conversion. Because of this, long-term use of lithium can result in hypothyroidism. Hypothyroidism, in turn, is linked to decreased serotonin levels and to depression, one of bipolar disorder's two components. Since lithium treatment generally is long-term, if you are taking lithium have your doctor check your blood thyroid levels every six months.

THYROID BALANCE AND
MIGRAINE HEADACHES

Thyroid imbalance and thyroid hormone supplements taken for underactive thyroid often take the blame for causing migraine headaches. For decades, doctors believed that migraine headaches were primarily vascular events, painful episodes caused by sudden variations in contraction and dilation of the arteries in the head. But now research seems to support what many people with thyroid imbalance have long believed: there is a link between thyroid function and migraine headache. The link even has a name: serotonin. That's right—the same neurotransmitter that regulates mood also seems to play a role in migraine headaches.

Migraines have long been linked to hormonal triggers. Many women who have PMS experience migraines during the week to ten days before their periods start. Older women who are transitioning to menopause might have cycles of migraine headaches that follow their changing hormone levels. Because hypothyroidism becomes significantly more common at menopause, the link between migraine, thyroid, and other hormones appears especially strong.

Restoring thyroid balance is of course important for overall health. Sometimes it is enough, by itself, to reduce the frequency and severity of migraines. But thyroid hormone supplement is not a treatment for migraine. When a migraine hits, most people need medications to relieve the pain and other symptoms. Nonsteroidal anti-inflammatory drugs (NSAIDs) such as ibuprofen or naproxen, are often effective because they reduce inflammation and swelling as well as relieve pain. These are available without a doctor's prescription.

There are a number of "migraine relief" products available over-the-counter in drugstores and grocery stores, too. Some of these include caffeine, which helps constrict blood vessels as well as potentiate (strengthen the effect of) the pain medication also in the product. Vitamin B_2 (riboflavin) and the herb feverfew both have been studied for their migraine-preventing effects. Look for a standardized extract form of feverfew; the plain herb will not work as well. For premenstrual or menstrual migraines, adjusting hormone levels with natural progesterone may be helpful. And magnesium, which has been shown to be depleted in the walls of vessels associated with migraines, can be used to treat an attack. Some doctors of natural medicine give monthly intravenous infusions of magnesium to their female patients who suffer from premenstrual migraines.

There are now prescription drugs available that can cut short a migraine before it gathers full momentum. Get a full workup and examination if you have migraines, however, before you start taking medications on your own. This will help identify any role your thyroid function is playing, and confirm that your symptoms are indeed caused by migraines.

18

Fertility, Thyroid, and a Woman's Cycle

Like so many other aspects of the human body's functions, fertility is an intricate and delicate balance. A wide range of hormones influences fertility both for men and for women. And it doesn't take much of a variation from what your body considers normal to upset the entire balance. Unlike other endocrine imbalances, however, with fertility you often don't know that an imbalance exists until you try to conceive.

THE HORMONES OF THE FERTILITY CYCLE

The hormones of the female fertility cycle involve multiple structures in the endocrine matrix. They include:

- Gonadotropin-releasing hormone (GnRH)—Directs pituitary to release FSH and LH
- Oxytocin—Causes uterus to contract during labor and childbirth
- Follicle-stimulating hormone (FSH)—Regulates egg production

- Luteinizing hormone (LH)—Regulates egg maturation and release (ovulation)
- Prolactin—Regulates milk production during and after pregnancy (lactation)
- Estrogen—Establishes female sex characteristics, regulates fertility cycle (we use the term "estrogen" as if this is a single hormone, but actually there are three estrogen hormones: estradiol, estrone, and estriol)
- Progesterone—Maintains environment in uterus to support pregnancy
- Testosterone—Affects sex drive, bone formation, and muscle strength
- Dehydroepiandrosterone (DHEA)—Reserve hormone of the adrenal gland that becomes progesterone, testosterone, or cortisol as needed.

During pregnancy, the levels of these hormones that are normally in the body change dramatically, and the placenta adds dozens more hormones to the mix.

THE CASCADE OF EVENTS

As a component of the endocrine matrix, the fertility cycle starts with the hypothalamus. The cascade of events that you know as your menstrual cycle starts deep within your brain, when your hypothalamus produces gonadotropin-releasing hormone (GnRH). GnRH directs the pituitary gland to produce follicle-stimulating hormone (FSH), which causes the ovaries to produce eggs. FSH also directs the ovaries to increase estrogen production, which in turn begins the process of carpeting the walls of the uterus with a thick network of blood vessels and tissue.

The rising estrogen levels signal your pituitary to cut back on the FSH, which tells the ovaries to cut estrogen production. At the same time, your pituitary releases luteinizing hormone

(LH), which causes your ovaries to release a mature egg from a follicle. This is the peak point of a woman's fertility cycle, ovulation. Once empty, the follicle produces both estrogen and progesterone.

Progesterone acts on the uterus to further thicken its lining, readying for a fertilized egg to implant. If this doesn't happen, the follicle stops its hormone production, causing both estrogen and progesterone levels to drop. The uterus can no longer sustain its enriched environment and begins to slough its lining, which passes out of the body through the vagina; this is menstruation. The average length of time it takes to complete this cycle is 28 days, but the range of normal is quite broad, from 21 to 35 days.

THE THYROID INFLUENCE

Thyroid hormone influences a woman's fertility in two ways. First, thyroid hormone regulates metabolism at the cell level in the ovaries, as it does throughout the body. When thyroid hormone levels are too low or too high, the altered metabolic rate interferes with the ability of ovarian cells to function properly. Fertility is such a carefully choreographed cascade of events that the tiniest misstep anywhere throws off the entire dance.

Second, estrogen, progesterone, and thyroid hormone are configured so that excess amounts of one can block the receptiveness of the cells to the others. In underactive thyroid, estrogen molecules tend to take up residence in available thyroid receptors. They have no action when they do this, but they do keep thyroid hormone molecules from binding with the receptors. This prevents thyroid hormone from playing its role in metabolism, further slowing cell functions. Oral contraceptive estrogens and estrogen replacement therapy also have this effect. In overactive thyroid, the opposite occurs. Thyroid hormone molecules bind to estrogen receptors in the cells. This keeps estrogen from binding, and interferes with the hormonal cycling of fertility.

When these disturbances remain relatively small-scale, they have little effect on the functions of either thyroid or estrogen. By the time thyroid imbalance becomes apparent (either through symptoms or blood test results), however, the consequence often shows as difficulty conceiving or carrying a pregnancy. Restoring thyroid balance restores fertility, to the extent that thyroid imbalance was the primary cause of the difficulties. Because fertility, like other endocrine cycles, is so complex, however, sometimes there are other factors involved that don't become apparent until thyroid balance is restored.

UNDERACTIVE THYROID AND FERTILITY

Some fertility experts believe that underactive thyroid in which blood thyroid levels are within normal ranges is a key factor among women who have trouble becoming pregnant. You might not even have obvious symptoms, and yet there's just enough of an imbalance present to interfere. If you are trying without success to conceive, make sure your doctor has done a complete thyroid panel (not just TSH and T4).

If your results are the slightest bit deviated from the normal ranges (and even if they're not, if you've taken other measures to improve your fertility without success), ask for a trial of treatment with thyroid hormone supplement. Some doctors use small doses of just T3, while others use low doses of levothyroxine. Check your blood thyroid levels in two weeks and in six weeks. If marginal hypothyroidism is present, you'll see at least small shifts in your levels and quite possibly a big shift in your fertility.

OVERACTIVE THYROID AND FERTILITY

Overactive thyroid that affects fertility usually shows its presence through blood tests. Drug therapy to restore thyroid balance—PTU or methimazole—doesn't usually interfere with fertility. Neither of these drugs is known to cause birth defects or problems with pregnancy, and doctors consider them safe to take. This is not the case with radioactive iodine therapy, however. If your doctor recommends I^{131} treatment to bring your thyroid function under control, don't try to conceive for at least three to six months following treatment. The potential for birth defects and other problems is high enough to be a concern. Your doctor is likely to suggest that you use a reliable form of birth control during treatment.

THYROID BALANCE DURING PREGNANCY

To say that pregnancy changes everything sounds at once trite and obvious. But "everything" runs the gamut from belly size to mitochondrial function. Metabolism revs up during pregnancy, so the woman's body can supply both the woman's and the baby's needs. Because metabolism is the domain of the thyroid, there are many changes that take place in thyroid function during pregnancy.

As we discussed in earlier chapters, thyroid hormone has two primary roles at the cell level. It permits production of long-term energy supplies (adenosine triphosphate—ATP), and it regulates production of short-term energy. When a woman's body is supporting another life, the need for both kinds of energy increases. A woman's metabolism increases by about 30 percent during pregnancy. The increased need for short-term energy is especially dramatic, since glucose fuels the baby's growth.

Thyroid hormone makes it possible for cells to increase their ability to combine oxygen and glucose to produce energy. The thyroid gland increases hormone production considerably to support this boost in energy production. Total T4 levels in the blood can double during pregnancy, increasing from the normal range of 5 to 12 micrograms/dl to 10 to 18 micrograms/dl. Since T4 is the body's storage form of thyroid hormone, this makes an abundant supply available to meet metabolic needs.

Other changes in thyroid balance take place, too. T4-to-T3 conversion increases, resulting in higher levels of total and free T3. The higher amounts of estrogen that are in a woman's body during pregnancy stimulate the liver to produce higher amounts of thyroid-binding globulin (TBG), which is why total T4 rises but free T4 decreases (the increased TBG binds with more T4). Of course, then, the drop in free T4 triggers the hypothalamus-pituitary response, which increases TSH to further stimulate the thyroid gland to increase hormone production. And the increased demand of the cells for more energy production (increased metabolism) stimulates increased conversion of T4 to T3, raising T3 levels as well.

During pregnancy, your entire endocrine matrix shifts. Other hormone balances also change. As the additional thyroid hormone in your blood increases cell metabolism, insulin production increases dramatically, too, to increase cell capacity for accepting glucose—another loop in the energy cycle.

The other component of thyroid balance during pregnancy is that of the fetus. Thyroid tissue arises early in development, and begins producing and secreting thyroid hormone by 12 weeks, although most of this is bound and so has no biological activity (as far as we know). Thyroid hormone is crucial for brain development. However, even though the fetus is producing its own thyroid hormone, most of its supply still comes from its mother. About 1 in 10,000 infants are born without a thyroid gland. As long as they receive immediate and ongoing thyroid hormone supplementation, this doesn't usually interfere with their development. In the United States, blood tests done at birth typically measure thyroid hormone levels.

OVERACTIVE THYROID IN PREGNANCY

The many shifts in hormone balances make it difficult to know when you're sliding into imbalance. Changing estrogen and progesterone levels cause many of the symptoms otherwise associated with hyperthyroidism. And metabolism is increased, so naturally there is evidence of that. Blood pressure, heart rate, and breathing rate all increase. You might feel flushed and unbearably hot one moment, then feel chilled the next. Symptoms such as tiredness, lack of energy, and rapid and wide mood swings are hallmarks of the first five months or so of pregnancy. Then hormone levels seem to stabilize for the next two or three months, and you might feel that you have an abundance of energy.

Hyperthyroidism is not very common in pregnancy, but it does occur. Typically, doctors check blood thyroid hormone levels at the first prenatal visit and then periodically during pregnancy. Your doctor is likely to order rechecks if you appear to have symptoms of overactive thyroid, just to be sure. Despite the initial perceptions of increased energy and stamina early in hyperthyroidism, overactive thyroid quickly becomes a drain on your body's resources.

Treatment for hyperthyroidism during pregnancy is usually propylthiouracil (PTU), which has few side effects and does not harm the fetus. Methimazole, the other drug therapy for hyperthyroidism, is more active when it crosses the placental barrier (moves from the mother's blood to the baby's blood). It doesn't appear to cause any problems, but doctors prefer to take the route of caution. Methimazole tends to cause more side effects in general among people who take it, so it is the drug of second choice anyway. Rarely, treatment with antithyroid drugs can cause underactive thyroid to be present in the baby at birth, but this almost always corrects itself within a few weeks. Blood tests done on the baby at birth will determine whether this is something that needs treatment.

Radioactive iodine therapy is *not* an option during pregnancy. I[131] does have action when it crosses the placental barrier, and would destroy the developing thyroid tissue. As well, the radioactive component raises the specter of birth defects because we know radiation causes alterations in genetic development. This is why doctors almost always order a pregnancy test before using I[131] treatment in a woman of childbearing age.

Nearly always, overactive thyroid during pregnancy returns to normal within weeks of delivery. Your doctor will monitor your blood thyroid hormone levels, and use them as guides for determining whether to continue antithyroid treatment. Often, you can stop the treatment as your body's overall hormonal balance returns to its prepregnancy state. When thyroid imbalance persists after delivery, it usually becomes postpartum hypothyroidism (more on this later in this chapter).

UNDERACTIVE THYROID IN PREGNANCY

Hypothyroidism already under control through thyroid hormone supplement therapy generally presents no problems during pregnancy, although you'll want to keep on top of your blood thyroid levels. It's not a bad idea to check them at least once per trimester. Your body's shifting hormonal balances, weight gain, and fluid retention—all of which occur normally during pregnancy—can change your body's need for thyroid hormone supplement, especially when coupled with your body's increasing demand for thyroid hormone. Your doctor might want to increase your supplement dose, add T3 to your therapy, or have an endocrinologist (physician who specializes in conditions involving the endocrine matrix) manage this dimension of your care during pregnancy.

Hypothyroidism that develops during pregnancy is more common than is hyperthyroidism, affecting about 1 in 100 pregnant women. Sometimes your thyroid gland just can't keep up with the demands your changing body is placing on it. Often, your thyroid balance was borderline before pregnancy, and is already at its maximum capacity to adjust. When this is the case, any major change in your body (such as illness, injury, or surgery) would be equally likely to set hypothyroidism in motion.

Again, it can be hard to separate some of the typical symptoms of pregnancy from those of thyroid imbalance. Tiredness, lack of energy, and mild fluid retention are common with both pregnancy and underactive thyroid. It becomes the subtle symptoms that are the tip-off that these could be the result of hypothyroidism. These symptoms are uniquely hypothyroidism:

- Dry, flaky, and even scaly skin, especially on the face, hands, and feet
- Brittle, coarse hair
- Hair loss, especially if in small, circular patches
- Loss of the outer portions of the eyebrows
- Hoarse voice
- Droopy eyelids and puffy eyes

Treatment for underactive thyroid during pregnancy is the same as when pregnancy is not a factor. Your body doesn't know the difference between thyroid hormone that comes from supplement and thyroid hormone that comes from your thyroid gland. Both affect cell metabolism in precisely the same ways. Because pregnancy intensifies the intricate balances of body systems, however, it is especially important that you take your thyroid supplement in the most effective ways.

- Take your thyroid hormone supplement at the same time every day. Try not to vary by more than 30 minutes. This helps maintain a consistent level of thyroid hormone in your bloodstream, stabilizing your endocrine matrix.

- Take your prenatal vitamins at least two hours (and preferably more) from the time you take your thyroid hormone supplement. Prenatal vitamins supply a high amount of iron because your body needs it, but iron binds to thyroid supplement, which prevents your body from using it.
- If you have morning sickness, take your thyroid supplement at a time of the day when nausea is least a problem. This helps assure that the maximum amount of thyroid hormone gets absorbed from your intestinal tract, particularly if vomiting accompanies the nausea. Many women experience nausea in the morning, giving rise to the term "morning sickness." But it can affect you at any time throughout the day or night.
- If you've been taking thyroid hormone supplement in the morning when you wake up but now you are nauseated at that time, switch your thyroid supplement to another time of the day and then stay with that schedule for the duration of your pregnancy. Throwing up every now and then after taking a thyroid dose isn't going to make a difference. If vomiting is a persistent problem, let your doctor know, because this can interfere with the absorption of nutrients, too.

Many women who develop hypothyroidism during pregnancy return to thyroid balance within weeks of delivery, and no longer need to take thyroid hormone supplement. Don't stop taking thyroid pills until your doctor tells you it's okay, though. Enough women continue to have thyroid imbalance after pregnancy that you should have your blood thyroid hormone levels checked two weeks, six weeks, and three months after delivery—whether or not you take thyroid hormone supplement during pregnancy. Some women develop postpartum thyroiditis or postpartum hypothyroidism after delivery; more on this later in this chapter.

MOTHER'S IMBALANCE: CRISIS FOR BABY?

Untreated hypothyroidism in the mom poses a significant threat for the baby. Proper brain development requires thyroid hormone. Although the fetus begins producing its own thyroid hormone early in development, only about 1 percent of that is active in the fetus's body. To meet most of its thyroid hormone needs, the fetus draws from its mother's supply. Numerous studies document delayed intellectual and emotional development in children born to mothers with untreated hypothyroidism, so this is a problem with serious ramifications for the child.

Another potential problem can arise even when a mother is being managed for hypothyroidism during pregnancy. During that pregnancy, the child is bathed in amniotic fluid that contains a fair amount of thyroid from the mother's medication. At birth, this suddenly is withdrawn. In a small number of newborns, this can lead to hypothyroidism at birth, as the infant's own thyroid gland struggles to keep thyroid levels up. For this reason, many obstetricians prefer to have a pediatric endocrinologist available at the childbirth of a woman with treated hypothyroidism.

THYROID IMBALANCE AND MISCARRIAGE

There is some evidence that untreated hypothyroidism in the mother makes miscarriage more of a risk. This is likely to be because of the interrelationships between thyroid hormone and estrogen and progesterone. The right balance between estrogen and progesterone is essential for maintaining a pregnancy. If that balance shifts beyond the usual changes that take place during pregnancy, the pregnancy is in jeopardy. Regular blood tests to assess thyroid function, as well as paying close attention to any symptoms that develop, can steer you to appropriate treatment early enough to avert this. Of course, not all miscarriages result from thyroid imbalance. But you want to address as many variables that are within your influence as you can, and thyroid balance is one of them. Thyroid hormone supplementation removes the risks of untreated hypothyroidism.

SOY INFANT FORMULA AND HYPOTHYROIDISM

In recent years, doctors have noticed an apparent connection between hypothyroidism in adolescents and adults and soy infant formula that they were fed as babies. Soy isoflavones, particularly genistein, have many effects on health. They are particularly powerful natural anticancer agents. But they seem to have a bit of a dark side when it comes to their influence on thyroid function. Soy can act as a potent thyroid suppressant, reducing the thyroid gland's production of thyroid hormone.

When they debuted several decades ago, soy infant formulas seemed the perfect alternative to milk-based formulas that often caused digestive problems because an infant's system isn't yet capable of digesting milk proteins. The chemical structures of human breast milk and cow's milk (from which milk-based infant formulas are derived) are close but not the same. Even removing some of the cow's-milk proteins during processing doesn't make them equitable. Not only can milk-based formulas be difficult for infants to digest, but also they can establish a lifetime of dairy allergy by activating antigens in the body. Iron deficiency also has been reported commonly in infants who drink a lot of cow's milk.

Soy-based infant formulas do not have these milk proteins. They are easy for babies to digest, and because they contain vitamin and mineral supplements, provide full nutrition for healthy growth and development. It's just now that the first generations of babies raised on soy infant formulas are coming to adulthood, which is why the possible connection between soy infant formula and hypothyroidism is just now becoming apparent. As yet health officials are not recommending that you avoid soy infant formulas, but this is likely to be a matter that gains significance as we learn more about the full extent of the risk.

One solution to this potential problem is for the manufacturers of soy infant formulas to remove the soy isoflavones from the products. Because soy infant formulas are so valuable in other ways, this seems a likely direction for manufacturers to take. However, soy isoflavone-free formulas are not yet on the market. Breastfeeding, of course, eliminates much of this problem. For any number of reasons, breastfeeding is recommended for at least a few months after childbirth.

POSTPARTUM HYPOTHYROIDISM

For reasons no one fully understands, some women develop hypothyroidism in the weeks and months following childbirth. Often this starts as hyperthyroidism and progresses to hypothyroidism. Postpartum hypothyroidism is an autoimmune condition in which your body develops antibodies that attack your thyroid tissue. At first this process stimulates thyroid hormone production, but then as thyroid tissue dies, hormone production drops.

Treatment is the same as for any other diagnosis of hypothyroidism—thyroid hormone supplement. About half of women who develop postpartum hypothyroidism find the condition to be temporary and are able to stop taking thyroid hormone supplement. For the other half, hypothyroidism is permanent and requires lifelong treatment. Doctors don't really know why this is. Women who have temporary hypothyroidism are more likely to develop hypothyroidism again later in life.

THYROID BALANCE AND PMS

Thyroid imbalance often exacerbates the symptoms of premenstrual syndrome (PMS). Because underactive thyroid often develops insidiously, you might notice worsening PMS before you recognize that your symptoms are also the same as those for underactive thyroid. If you already take thyroid hormone supplement and are having trouble managing your PMS, ask your doctor to check your blood thyroid levels to make sure your dose is optimal.

Many herbal products for PMS and women's health maintenance contain high amounts of soy isoflavones and phytoestrogens (plant-based estrogens). Although these are often helpful in smoothing the ups and downs of estrogen and progesterone levels during your monthly cycles, when taken in excessively high doses they can have the effect of suppressing thyroid function. This can result in temporary hypothyroidism. Usually, cutting back on the herbal products will ease this effect, allowing thyroid function to return to normal.

THYROID BALANCE AND BIRTH CONTROL PILLS

Thyroid hormone supplement interacts with the estrogen in birth control pills, causing less of the estrogen to enter your bloodstream. Many women see an endocrinologist, internist, or family practitioner for care related to thyroid, but go to a gynecologist for needs such as contraception. Be sure the doctor who prescribes your birth control pills knows that you take thyroid hormone supplement. Generally, doctors prescribe oral contraceptives with a higher amount of estrogen to offset the interaction with thyroid hormone supplement. The "low hormone" birth control pills may not be a good choice if you take thyroid hormone supplement.

THYROID BALANCE AND MENOPAUSE

The likelihood of thyroid imbalance increases as you get older. For women, this can mean a collision between thyroid and menopause. The general symptoms of each are similar: fatigue, changes in hair and skin, trouble sleeping, anxiety, depression, heart palpitations, and missed periods. But there are distinctive symptoms that can help separate the two.

Symptoms of Thyroid Imbalance vs. Menopause	
Symptoms Likely to Be Thyroid Imbalance	Symptoms Likely to Be Menopause
Neck pain	Hot flashes
Swelling in arms and legs	Night sweats
Losing eyebrows or eyelashes	Vaginal dryness
Significant weight gain or loss	Modest, gradual weight gain

An easy way to distinguish between thyroid imbalance and menopause is to have blood tests done to measure your thyroid hormone levels and your FSH level. FSH rises with menopause, as estrogen levels drop. Menopause and thyroid imbalance tend to intensify each other's symptoms.

Soy isoflavones have become popular for their ability to reduce some of the discomforts of menopause. But these substances are also thyroid suppressants—they decrease thyroid function. If you are taking soy-based products for menopause symptoms and find that the symptoms seem to be getting worse instead of better, it could be that the cause is thyroid imbalance rather than menopause.

THYROID BALANCE AND SEXUAL FUNCTION

There's no escaping the endocrine matrix when it comes to hormonal balance. When your thyroid is out of balance, so are your other hormones—including sex hormones. Underactive thyroid is linked with premature ejaculation in men, inability to reach orgasm in women, and low libido (sex drive) in both men and women. As is the case with most of underactive thyroid's symptoms, restoring thyroid balance generally eliminates these problems.

Knowledge about the connection between thyroid balance and sexual function has been limited until recent research began establishing the links. Much of the connection relates to thyroid's role in cell metabolism; sluggish cells just don't function at optimal levels, and this affects many body systems. There also is evidence that underactive thyroid interferes with sperm production in men, possibly affecting fertility.

19

Energy in Balance: Getting into a Healthy Synchronicity

When you have a thyroid imbalance, ongoing medical care becomes a necessary element of your health and your life. If you have underactive thyroid, you will need to take thyroid hormone supplement for the rest of your life, barring technological advances that give us new ways to approach and treat thyroid dysfunction (which might not be all that far off). Accept these treatments and the help that they give your body. But don't ignore alternatives that can enhance your conventional treatment.

The previous 18 chapters are all about balance within and among the matrixes, systems, structures, and chemicals of your body. This reflects the Western perspective of balance: focus on the parts to align the whole. The Eastern perspective takes the converse view: focus on the whole, and the parts will align themselves. Whether your thyroid is underactive or overactive, and whatever path of treatment you choose from conventional medicine, the philosophies and practices of the Eastern perspective are certain to help you feel more calm, centered, and, yes, balanced.

LIFE IS ENERGY

In the Eastern view, prana is the universal energy. Prana, like the air we breathe, is all around us. It gives life. Qi (pronounced "chee" and sometimes spelled ki or chi) is the energy of your body. It flows through you, sustaining and connecting the vital components of body, mind, and spirit. When there is health and balance among these components, there is health. When one is out of balance, all are out of balance. It is affected by diet and lifestyle factors, by genetics, and by emotions. Sound familiar? It's a matrixlike concept, not all that different from the concept of matrix that provides a framework for understanding the intricate interrelationships of thyroid function.

As a structure of the physical world, the human body is an amalgam of electrons and neutrons. This gives the body polarity, just like a magnet—just like all structures of the physical world. Electrical and magnetic energies are constantly active in your body, and make possible the multitude of chemical and physical interactions that constitute life. The first medical technology to take advantage of these energies was the electrocardiogram (ECG), developed in the early 1900s. ECG captures electrical impulses of the heart and converts them to written signals that doctors use to interpret heart function. Following in the ECG's shadow was the x-ray, which combined knowledge of atom-level structure, just evolving in the early 1900s, and very-short-wave electromagnetic radiation. Through the decades of the twentieth century, this basic technology evolved into an entire field of practice called nuclear medicine. And in the 1970s came magnetic resonance imaging (MRI), which uses the body's magnetic field to form pictures of organs and body structures, soft tissue and bone. For over a hundred years now, medical technology had made use of the body's energy fields to diagnose and treat illnesses.

Of course, this pales in comparison to traditional Chinese medicine (TCM) and other Eastern healing systems, which have used the body's energy fields for diagnosis and healing, albeit not in such technological ways, for nearly 5,000 years!

QI: THE BODY'S ENERGY

Qi, the energy that sustains your body and its functions, exists in two complementing forms, yin and yang. Yin energy is characterized as cool, moist, passive, dark, and feminine. It is structure, solid, and can be measured. It is symbolized by the Earth. Yang energy represents warm, dry, active, light, and masculine. It is movement, and functional rather than structural. It is symbolized by the heavens, which are immeasurable. In health, yin and yang exist in balance. It is a dynamic balance, ever shifting back and forth from yin dominance to yang dominance. When either yin or yang remains in dominance, however, the other is inadequate and a state of imbalance—unhealth—results.

Conceptually, this is quite similar to the Western view of homeostasis, or the balance of function within the human body. Many of these functions exist in complementary pairings—you breathe in, you breathe out. Your heart's atria (upper chambers) draw blood in, its ventricles (lower chambers) pump blood out. Even the balances of your endocrine matrix exist in cycles of complementary activity, with many hormones paired for their opposite activities (insulin lowers blood sugar, glucagons raises it, and parathyroid hormone increases blood calcium while calcitonin lowers it). In other examples, low levels of hormones initiate certain sequences and high levels of hormones initiate other sequences.

Qi, which is not visible, comes from two sources, the life energy that is yours from birth and the energy you put into your body through the prana (air) that you breathe and the foods that you eat. Qi flows through your body via a network of unseen channels called meridians. Meridians roughly coincide with the structures of your nervous system, although they don't have a physical structure. There are 12 primary (sometimes called major) meridians that occur in pairs and 8 secondary (sometimes called minor) meridians. The inner, or central, meridians flow upward and carry yin energy; the outer, or lateral, meridians flow downward and carry yang energy.

The primary meridians correspond to your body's major organs: heart, lungs, liver, kidneys, spleen, bladder, gallbladder, stomach, large intestine, small intestine, and two functions not recognized in Western physiology, the pericardium and the triple burner. The pericardium encircles your heart energy much as your physical pericardium encloses your heart, and its role is similarly protective, but of the flow of energy rather than the flow of blood. The triple burner regulates and distributes energy and heat through the three zones of your body: upper, middle, and lower. In a general way (and remembering that this is not a physical structure), its functions resemble those of your thyroid gland.

The primary meridians circulate qi to your body's organs. When qi becomes blocked, the point of blockage determines the affected organs. Those that relate to the endocrine matrix directly are shown on page 276.

The secondary meridians carry qi that supports your emotional, psychological, and spiritual health. Blockages in the secondary meridians affect your mood, thought processes, memory, and overall sense of well-being.

Qi can be augmented, and moved through the body in a number of ways. Acupuncture utilizes thin needles in points along the meridians. Sometimes, the needles are heated, or heat is applied directly through the burning of an herb called "moxa" to warm a point. In recent years, electrical stimulation, magnets, and lasers have been used to address qi during an acupuncture treatment.

Qi Blockage and Associated Imbalance		
Organ	Relationship or Function	Imbalance Associated With
Heart	immune system	frequent infections, autoimmune disorders
Spleen and liver	process the energy that enters your body as food and distribute it to replenish your qi	worry and anxiety, energy imbalances throughout the body
Bladder and kidneys	autonomic nervous system, sex drive, warmth	inflammation, exhaustion, chronic fatigue syndrome

Chinese herbs are also used to unblock qi that is stuck, and to build qi that is deficient. In Chinese herbal medicine, the herbs are given in formulas of 6–20 herbs that work synergistically to balance the yin and yang in the meridians. In this way it is different from Western herbal medicine, in which specific herbs are given for specific effects on diseases or organs.

QIGONG

Chinese herbal medicine and acupuncture require a licensed, experienced practitioner. What can you do yourself to improve your thyroid condition, and your health generally, by improving the movement of your qi? For this, the ancient Chinese developed a system called QiGong, literally "energy exercises." Most martial arts (like kung fu and karate) are actually forms of QiGong. The simplest form of QiGong is the standing QiGong.

Chinese medicine was developed eons before the thyroid gland was known to be in the neck, and so there are not specific treatments for thyroid problems. But, there is a channel of energy called the Triple Warmer that has to do with temperature regulation, and another called the Spleen that has to do with metabolism. QiGong exercises for the Spleen and Triple Warmer are simple. Because the Triple Warmer refers to the three cavities of the body whose heat needs to be balanced (chest, abdomen, pelvis), Triple Warmer QiGong moves qi into these areas.

- Stand with feet shoulder-length apart, knees slightly bent.
- Sweep both hands in front of you, chest high, as if gathering in the air toward your chest.
- Repeat this motion seven times, gathering qi into the abdomen, and seven times into the pelvis.

This brings qi into each of the three cavities, and strengthens the Triple Warmer.

YOGA: JOINING BODY, MIND, AND SPIRIT

Yoga is another approach to rebalancing qi. The word yoga means "to yoke" or to unite. Yoga uses a blend of physical poses and meditation to join your physical, mental, and spiritual energies. Some poses target specific organs or systems, and others rebalance the body in whole. Yoga activates the structures of your energy system called chakras. You have seven chakras, each of which corresponds to a physical location and a structure of your endocrine matrix. They are the following.

Chakra	Physical Location	Endocrine Structure Affiliation
Root (first)	Base of the spine	Sex glands (ovaries or testes)
Spleen (second)	Sex organs	Pancreas
Solar plexus (third)	Solar plexus (mid-abdomen)	Adrenal glands
Heart (fourth)	Heart (mid-chest)	Thymus gland
Throat (fifth)	Base of the neck	Thyroid gland
Brow (sixth; also called "third eye")	Center of the forehead	Pituitary gland
Crown (seventh)	Top of the head	Pineal gland

As you can see, the direct correlation to thyroid function is the throat chakra. Yoga postures that stimulate the throat chakra help to restore energy balance (not necessarily hormonal) to the thyroid gland. And as you know by this point in the book, all of your endocrine structures and their functions are inseparably intertwined. Yoga postures that stimulate any of the chakras help to restore energy balance all along your endocrine matrix.

YOGA BREATHING

Prana is the essence of life energy, and breathing to bring it into your body is the essence of yoga. Prana replenishes and revitalizes qi. Yoga breathing techniques help you to bring prana into your body. The following are some basic yoga breathing techniques.

- Drawing breath—take in a slow, long breath through your nose. Consciously feel the energy of this breath fill your lungs, see it flow through your body.
- Extending breath—let your breath out in a slow, long, smooth exhale through your nose. Consciously feel its energy return to the air.
- Warming breath—breathe in and out, sharply but deeply, through your nose, using your diaphragm for power and control. Feel your belly button move in with each inhale and out with each exhale, and feel each breath fill your body with warmth and energy.
- Cooling breath—open your lips slightly. Draw in a breath as though sucking from a straw, slowly and steadily. Feel the breath fill your lungs and your body. Hold the breath for a few seconds, and then let it out slowly through your nose.

As they replenish your qi, breathing techniques improve the energy balance of your body overall.

YOGA POSTURES

Yoga postures are physical positions that direct energy toward certain chakras and away from others. Yoga postures should never hurt! You might feel a stretch, but you should never push until you feel pain. The best way to learn yoga is to take a class from a qualified instructor. If you have any health conditions that limit your strength or flexibility, discuss them with the instructor so he or she can help you modify yoga postures in ways that allow you to do them with maximum benefit. If you are unsure whether your yoga practice will interfere with your health conditions, check with your doctor before you start doing yoga.

The postures that release each chakra are too numerous to mention here (see Appendix B for yoga resources). Two postures that activate your chakras in general are the prana arch and the open pose. The prana arch releases the chakras in the chest and throat, and the open pose releases the chakras in the abdomen and pelvis. Both improve the flow of prana through all of the chakras.

Prana Arch

- Stand with your hands at your sides, feet about shoulder-width apart and eyes looking straight out.
- Inhale slowly, and as you do, pull your head up as if looking toward the ceiling.
- At the same time, raise your hands, palms outward, up and out from your shoulders.
- Allow yourself to lean backward as far as is comfortable. Breathe slowly and deeply, in and out, for several breaths.
- Exhale a last time, slowly, and lower your arms and your head.

Open Pose

For this pose, you need one to three pillows.

- Lie on the floor on your back, with your head on a pillow.
- Bring the soles of your feet together so they are touching. Lower your knees to the floor on either side (use a pillow to support each knee if this is awkward or uncomfortable).
- Touch your palms together, and rest them on your chest at your heart chakra.
- Breathe in and out, slowly and deeply. Feel the breath fill your lungs and your body.
- Continue until you feel relaxed and energized. Move slowly and smoothly to release from this pose.

YOGA FOR THYROID BALANCE: THE SHOULDER POSE

One yoga posture, the shoulder pose or shoulder stand, is specifically for the thyroid. This pose requires a greater degree of strength, flexibility, and balance than the prana arch and the open pose. Move slowly and smoothly as you do this pose. If it feels uncomfortable, stop. With practice, you'll get better.

- Start by lying flat on your back on the floor, legs together and straight out, arms flat at your sides and your palms facing down.
- Breathe in and out, slowly and with purpose.
- Bring your knees to your chest so that your thighs are pressing your abdomen.
- Put your hands under your hips for support, and smoothly raise your trunk until it is perpendicular with the floor. Move your hands up your lower back to provide continued support. Eventually your chin will touch your chest.
- Extend your legs so they are straight out and also perpendicular to the floor. Keep them together, and point your toes.
- Breathe slowly and smoothly, feeling your breath fill your lungs and your body.
- Hold the pose for as long as it feels comfortable. Feel the energy flow to your throat and torso.
- To release the pose, slowly reverse your movements. Bring your legs down so your thighs are touching your abdomen, then lower your trunk until your hips are again on the floor. Extend your legs out flat, and bring your arms down to your sides.

The shoulder pose activates the throat chakra, flooding it with energy.

MINDFUL AWARENESS: MEDITATION

Meditation is an excellent technique to relieve stress and restore a sense of vitality to your body, mind, and spirit. There are many forms of meditation (again, Appendix B provides some resources to get you started). If you're not accustomed to meditating, you might wonder how it's possible to empty your mind of thought. This isn't really the point! Rather than clearing your mind, most forms of meditation instead focus on filling your mind with a single thought, image, or sound. This calms and quiets your busy brain, bringing renewed energy and relieving stress.

Here is a basic meditation:

- Find a quiet location where you won't be disturbed for 5 to 10 minutes.
- Take a comfortable, open position. Some people sit, others lie down. Just make sure your arms and legs are open (don't cross them).
- Close your eyes to help focus your attention inward.
- Take three slow, deep breaths. Feel the breath fill your lungs, and expanding from your abdomen to your chest and reaching out through your entire body.
- Select an image, thought, or sound to focus on. This can be just about anything, but try to keep it simple. If you can't think of anything on your own to start with, use the image of a butterfly.
- See the butterfly enter your mind. Watch how its wings move. Observe its colors and textures. See where the wings attach to the body. Look at the delicate, threadlike legs.
- Gradually narrow your focus to the largest spot of color on the butterfly's left wing. Let the color fill your mind. See nothing but the color, see everything about the color.

- Gradually widen your focus again. See the color again become a spot on the butterfly's wing. See the other wing, and the whole butterfly. Watch it begin to flutter its wings, preparing to take off.
- As the butterfly lifts into flight, envision that it pulls with it a nearly invisible and extraordinarily light string. Attached to this string are your worries, fears, concerns, cares. Watch the butterfly as it disappears, pulling away the thoughts that cause tension and stress.
- Take three slow, deep breaths. Feel the breaths fill your lungs and your body.
- Open your eyes, and let yourself see the beauty and calm that surrounds you.

INTEGRATING EAST WITH WEST

Health is about balance, synergy, and synchronicity. One thing leads to another . . . to another . . . to another. Always.

Not all Eastern approaches will appeal to you or work for you. Just as you must find the treatments that are right for you in conventional, or Western, medicine, you must find the Eastern approaches that are right for you. The therapies of Eastern medicine are entirely compatible with the treatments of Western medicine. When you integrate the two, you establish for yourself a true environment of balance . . . in thyroid function, within your metabolic matrix, in health, and in life. Equilibrium heals and replenishes all.

Glossary

Achilles tendon reflex test—measurement of how rapidly the Achilles tendon contracts the calf muscle upon stimulation; a test of thyroid function from before the time of blood tests that is enjoying a resurgence of popularity as an additional diagnostic tool in identifying thyroid imbalance particularly when blood-test results appear normal or are inconclusive

acupuncture—healing system based in traditional Chinese medicine (TCM) that redirects the flow of energy through very thin, flexible needles inserted into the skin at specific locations

Addison's disease—condition in which damage to the adrenal glands prevents them from producing cortisol and other hormones; often an autoimmune condition

adrenal fatigue—condition in which the adrenal glands function in a constant "stress response" mode and adrenal hormones in the body become imbalanced

adrenal glands—pair of glands located on the tops of the kidneys, responsible for producing stress hormones and other hormones

adrenocorticotropic hormone (ACTH)—hormone the pituitary gland produces that directs the adrenal glands to release cortisol

aldosterone—hormone the adrenal glands produce that regulates sodium elimination by the kidneys

alopecia areata—autoimmune condition in which hair comes out in circular patches. When associated with hypothyroidism, the hair can return when hypothyroidism is treated

antidiuretic hormone (ADH)—hormone the hypothalamus produces that regulates the fluid retention functions of the kidneys

antithyroglobulin antibodies—immune proteins that attack the protein that binds with T3 and T4. When present in the body they suggest an autoimmune thyroid disorder such as Graves' disease or Hashimoto's thyroiditis

antithyroid drugs—drugs that destroy thyroid tissue to reduce its production of thyroid hormone; treatment for hyperthyroidism

antithyroid microsomal antibodies—immune proteins present in the body that attack the cells of the thyroid gland. When present, they suggest an autoimmune thyroid disorder such as Graves' disease or Hashimoto's thyroiditis

antithyroperoxidase (anti-TPO) antibodies—immune proteins that attack a thyroid-related enzyme. When present in the blood they indicate an autoimmune thyroid disorder such as Graves' disease or Hashimoto's thyroiditis; more sensitive than other antibody tests

apathetic hyperthyroidism—form of overactive thyroid that shows symptoms similar to hypothyroidism; more common in elderly people

Armour Thyroid—brand of natural desiccated thyroid

autoimmune disorder—condition in which the body's immune system attacks a particular organ or structure in the body, viewing it as an invader that must be destroyed

B cells—cells of the immune system that come to maturity in the bone marrow and produce and carry antibodies

basal body temperature—body temperature at rest, usually taken immediately upon waking using a thermometer placed under the arm (axillary temperature); sometimes called the Broda Barnes method of diagnosing thyroid imbalance; when taken by mouth, it measures core basal body temperature, which is not as good an indicator of thyroid function

beta blockers—drugs that control the body's "fight-or-flight" response to reduce symptoms of hyperthyroidism such as rapid heart rate and breathing, sweating, and feelings of anxiety; these drugs have no direct effect on thyroid function

biopsy—diagnostic procedure in which cells are removed from the thyroid gland and examined under a microscope to determine whether they are cancerous

body mass index (BMI)—means of assessing what relationship exists between body weight and health problems

bound T3—T3 in circulation in the body that is attached to protein; considered biologically inactive; term also identifies the blood test that measures the amount of bound T3 in the blood

bound T4—T4 in circulation in the body that is attached to protein; considered biologically inactive; term also identifies the blood test that measures the amount of bound T4 in the blood

cholesterol—form of fatty acid present in some foods and also in the human body, where it is used to produce the steroid stress hormones and sex hormones

chronic fatigue syndrome—collection of symptoms marked by overwhelming tiredness; sometimes linked to hypothyroidism, low adrenal function, and weakened immune system

cognition—activities of thinking, reasoning, and memory that take place in the brain

congenital hypothyroidism—disorder that occurs when a baby is born without a thyroid gland or fails to receive enough dietary iodine for its thyroid gland to make thyroid hormone, resulting in severe or complete lack of thyroid hormone in the body; when not treated, results in permanent brain damage and stunted physical growth

corticotropin-releasing hormone (CRH)—hormone the hypothalamus produces that directs the pituitary gland to release ACTH

cortisol—hormone the adrenal glands produce in response to stress; it maintains blood pressure, aids metabolism, and reduces inflammation (also called hydrocortisone)

cretinism—old word used to describe the constellation of symptoms, including severe mental retardation, accompanying what is now called congenital hypothyroidism

Cytomel—brand of drug containing T3 supplement (liothyronine)

dehydroepiandrosterone (DHEA)—hormone the adrenal glands produce that acts as a reserve for other hormones and plays a role in mitigating the effects of stress and aging

deoxyribonucleic acid (DNA)—molecule in the nuclei of all cells; it contains genetic information

diabetes (diabetes mellitus)—endocrine disorder in which the pancreas stops producing insulin (type 1 diabetes) or cells in the body become resistant to insulin (type 2 diabetes); type 1 is a known autoimmune disorder; some forms of type 2 are suspected to be autoimmune as well

diiolo-L-thyronine (T2)—form of thyroid hormone whose action is not yet well understood but appears to play a role in mitochondrial binding and metabolism

endocrine matrix—network of structures and functions that form the endocrine system

endocrine organ—an organ that produces a substance called a hormone that is secreted directly into the blood stream

epinephrine—hormone (also called a neurotransmitter) the adrenal glands produce that raises blood pressure, heart rate, and blood sugar level as part of the body's "fight-or-flight" response to stress

erythrocyte—red blood cell

estrogen—hormone the ovaries (and, to a lesser extent, the adrenal glands and fat cells) produce that directs female sex characteristics and regulates a woman's fertility cycle; present in males in small amounts

euthyroid—state of normal thyroid function and balance

euthyroid sick syndrome—condition in which severe trauma alters thyroid function without altering thyroid production of thyroid hormone

exocrine gland—organ that produces substances, such as saliva and digestive enzymes, that are secreted through ducts to where in the body they have their activity

fatigue—extreme and long-lasting tiredness that interferes with daily functions

fibromyalgia—chronic condition marked by muscle and joint pain, extreme fatigue, and sleep disturbances; frequently develops after an injury, illness, or traumatic situation

follicle-stimulating hormone (FSH)—hormone the pituitary gland produces that directs the ovaries to produce eggs in women and the testes to produce sperm in men

free T3—biologically active form of T3 in circulation in the body that is not bound to protein; term also identifies the blood test that measures the amount of free T3 in the blood

free T4—biologically active form of T4 in circulation in the body that is not bound to protein; term also identifies the blood test that measures the amount of free T4 in the blood

glucagon—hormone the pancreas produces that increases blood sugar levels in response to the body's demands for energy

goiter—swelling of the thyroid gland; can appear with hypothyroidism or hyperthyroidism; diffuse goiter involves swelling of the entire thyroid gland; multinodular goiter involves swelling of localized areas

goitrogenic foods—foods, such as soy and cruciferous vegetables, that interfere with the thyroid gland's ability to absorb iodine

gonadotropin-releasing hormone (GnRH)—hormone the hypothalamus produces that directs the pituitary gland to release FSH and LH

Graves' disease—autoimmune disorder involving the thyroid gland; most common form of hyperthyroidism; also called diffuse toxic goiter

Hashimoto's thyroiditis—autoimmune disorder that results in hypothyroidism; accounts for about 80 percent of hypothyroidism cases; sometimes starts as hyperthyroidism

heart palpitations—feeling that your heart is pounding so hard and fast that it is going to come out of your chest

high-sensitivity thyroid-stimulating hormone assay (TSH or sTSH assay)—very sensitive blood test to measure the amount of thyroid-stimulating hormone in the blood

hormone—chemical that an endocrine structure produces that carries chemical messages throughout your body

HPA axis—matrix of the hypothalamus, pituitary gland, and adrenal glands and their interrelated functions

HPT axis—matrix of the hypothalamus, pituitary gland, and the thyroid gland and their interrelated functions

Human Genome Project (HGP)—collaborative scientific effort to identify and map the entire sequence of genetic information that defines the human being

human growth hormone (HGH)—hormone the pituitary gland produces that regulates childhood growth and muscle strength in adulthood; also raises blood sugar; thought by some to have a critical role in the aging process

hyperthyroid—circumstance of having excess thyroid function

hypothalamus—endocrine structure located in the center of the brain that is "command central" for the endocrine matrix

hypothyroid—circumstance of having inadequate thyroid function

infiltrative dermopathy—condition associated with Graves' disease in which lesions form on the skin of the shins; an autoimmune disorder that runs a course separate from Graves' disease once it develops

infiltrative ophthalmopathy—condition involving the structures surrounding the eyes in Graves' disease; symptoms include "bulging" eyes and weakness in the muscles that control eye movement; an autoimmune disorder that runs a course separate from Graves' disease once it develops

inhibin—hormone the testes produce that regulates sperm production

insulin—hormone the pancreas produces that regulates glucose use at the cell level and maintains blood glucose balance; when elevated, has adverse effects on weight, immunity, and cardiovascular system

iodine—naturally occurring element that the thyroid gland uses (in combination with the protein tyrosine) to make thyroid hormone

iodized salt—table salt to which iodine has been added as a means to ensure that people get enough dietary iodine to support proper thyroid function

leukocyte—white blood cell

Levothroid—brand of levothyroxine (synthetic T4 supplement)

levothyroxine—synthetic form of thyroxine (T4), taken as a thyroid hormone supplement

Levoxyl—brand of levothyroxine (synthetic T4 supplement)

Liotrix—brand of thyroid hormone supplement that contains a combination of synthetic T4 (levothyroxine) and synthetic T3 (liothyronine)

luteinizing hormone (LH)—hormone the pituitary gland produces that regulates egg maturation and release in women and directs the testes to release testosterone in men

lymph—watery fluid that circulates through your lymphatic system; carries lymphocytes (specialized infection-fighting white blood cells) and proteins; removes waste products from the tissues

melanocyte-stimulating hormone (MSH)—hormone the pituitary gland produces that directs the skin cells to darken pigment

melatonin—hormone the pineal gland produces that regulates the sleep cycle

menopause—name given to the end of a woman's years of fertility cycles

metabolic matrix—network or web of body structures and activities related to the functions of living; includes the influences of external environment, internal environment, and the constant communication among body organs

metabolism—the functions of living

methimazole—antithyroid drug

mitochondrion—place within the cell where most metabolism occurs

myxedema—old term for hypothyroidism that refers to the facial swelling that often accompanies underactive thyroid

myxedemic coma—rare but life-threatening crisis in untreated hypothyroidism in which the body has virtually no circulating thyroid hormone and begins to shut down; with emergency treatment, recovery is usually complete

natural desiccated thyroid—thyroid supplement prepared from dried and purified tissue from animal (usually pig) thyroid glands

neurotransmitters—chemicals the body produces that facilitate communication among nerve cells and between nerve cells and other cells

nodule—lump or swelling in the thyroid gland; more than 95 percent of nodules are noncancerous

norepinephrine—hormone (also called a neurotransmitter) the adrenal glands produce that raises blood pressure; part of the body's "fight-or-flight" response

nutritional supplement—vitamin, mineral, or other natural product available for general purchase and use without a prescription; does not contain a drug

osteoporosis—condition in which the bones lose calcium, weakening them and making them vulnerable to fracture

ovaries—female sex glands; produce sex hormones and eggs

overactive thyroid—casual term for hyperthyroidism; exists when the thyroid gland produces too much thyroid hormone

oxytocin—hormone the hypothalamus produces that causes the uterus to contract during labor and childbirth

pancreas—endocrine gland that produces insulin and glucagon; also is an exocrine gland, producing digestive enzymes

parathyroid glands—collection of four glands loosely attached to the thyroid gland; produce parathyroid hormone

parathyroid hormone—hormone the parathyroid glands produce that regulates the body's calcium and phosphate levels

peripheral T4-to-T3 conversion—process that takes place within the liver and other tissues in which circulating T4 loses an iodine atom and becomes T3; under some circumstances it becomes reverse T3 (rT3), a less active substance

pineal gland—endocrine structure located deep within the brain; involved in regulating day-night and other circadian cycles

pituitary gland—structure of the endocrine matrix that is in the brain beneath the hypothalamus; sometimes called "master gland" for its control functions of other glands

placenta—an organ that develops during pregnancy to support the developing fetus

polyglandular deficiency syndrome—condition in which multiple structures of the endocrine matrix function improperly

postpartum hypothyroidism—underactive thyroid that develops in a woman following pregnancy

primary thyroid dysfunction—problems with thyroid function that occur as a result of dysfunction within the thyroid gland itself

progesterone—hormone the ovaries produce that directs blood vessel growth in the uterus, in preparation for pregnancy, as part of a woman's monthly fertility cycle

prolactin—hormone the pituitary gland produces that directs the breasts to produce milk during and after pregnancy

propylthiouracil (PTU)—antithyroid drug

qi—(in Eastern practices such as TCM), refers to life energy that flows through all living things

radioactive iodine—iodine molecules that contain radiation, usually I[131]

radioactive iodine uptake (RAUI)—test that uses radioactive iodine to measure how much iodine the thyroid gland absorbs; uses imaging technology to present a dimensional scan of the thyroid gland; done to assess whether the thyroid gland is capable of making thyroid hormone

radioimmunoassay (RIA)—sophisticated method for measuring thyroid hormones in the blood

resin T3 uptake—blood test done in conjunction with total T3 to determine whether variations in total T3 are the result of altered thyroid function or thyroid binding

resin T4 uptake—blood test done in conjunction with total T4 to determine whether variations in total T4 are the result of altered thyroid function or thyroid binding

reverse T3 (rT3)—an inactive form of T3 that slows metabolism; term also identifies the blood test that measures the amounts of rT3 in the body

rheumatoid arthritis—autoimmune disorder in which the body develops antibodies that attack the joints; progressive, can be painful and deforming

secondary thyroid dysfunction—problems with thyroid function that arise as the result of other health conditions

serum thyroxine level—also called total thyroxine, total T4, or T4; blood test that measures the total amount of T4, free and bound, in the blood

serum triiodothyronine—also called total T3; blood test that measures the total amount of T3, free and bound, in the blood

sex glands—collective term for ovaries (women) and testes (men)

subclinical—a condition that exists when there is clinical evidence of it but no symptoms

Synthroid—levothyroxine; first synthetic T4 supplement on the market and the most commonly prescribed such product on the market today

T2—see diiolo-L-thyronine

T3—see triiodothyronine

T4—see thyroxine

T cells—cells of the immune system that come to maturity in the thymus and attack antigens (foreign proteins)

testes—male sex glands; produce sex hormones and sperm

testosterone—hormone the testes produce that directs male sex characteristics and causes sperm to mature; also produced in the ovaries, affecting sexual response and lubrication in women

thymosin—hormone the thymus produces that directs immune system development in children

thymus gland—endocrine structure located in the middle of the chest; responsible for immune system T-cell programming; diminishes in size in adulthood

thyroglobulin—protein that binds with T4 and T3

thyroid-binding globulin (TBG)—test that measures the amount of thyroid-binding globulin, the protein structure that binds with T3 and T4, in the blood

thyroid gland—butterfly-shaped endocrine structure that lies across the front of the neck just below the Adam's apple

thyroidectomy—surgical removal of part or all of the thyroid gland

thyroid hormone supplement—drug taken to supplement or replace the body's thyroid hormone

thyroiditis—inflammation of the thyroid gland

thyroid resistance—state in which the thyroid gland does not respond properly to thyroid hormone supplement

thyroid-stimulating hormone (TSH)—hormone the pituitary gland produces that directs the thyroid to release T3 and T4

thyroid storm—sudden and potentially life-threatening attack of hyperthyroidism that requires emergency treatment; recovery is usually complete with treatment; also called thyrotoxic crisis

thyroid ultrasound—test using ultrasound (high-frequency sound waves) that creates a dimensional image of the thyroid gland to identify nodules and cysts

Thyroid USP—generic brand of natural desiccated thyroid

thyrotoxicosis factitiae—overdose of thyroid hormone from taking too much thyroid hormone supplement; produces symptoms of hyperthyroidism but not the typical pattern of blood-test results

thyrotropin-releasing hormone (TRH)—hormone the hypothalamus produces that directs the pituitary gland to release TSH

thyroxine (T4)—long-acting hormone the thyroid gland produces that directs cellular metabolism; also serves as storehouse for conversion to T3 as needed; active ingredient in synthetic thyroid hormone supplement products such as Synthroid (levothyroxine)

toxic nodular goiter—localized swelling in the thyroid gland that causes overproduction of thyroid hormone

Traditional Chinese medicine (TCM)—system of healing and balance that forms the basis of Chinese herbal medicine and acupuncture; several thousand years old

TRH stimulation—test to determine whether the pituitary gland is appropriately releasing thyroid-stimulating hormone

triiodothyronine (T3)—short-acting hormone the thyroid gland produces that directs cellular metabolism; active ingredient in the T3 supplement product Cytomel

TSH by IRMA—thyroid-stimulating hormone measured by immunoradiometric assay; very sensitive test that measures the amounts of TSH in the blood as they rise and fall in response to the amounts of T3 and T4 in the blood

tyrosine—amino acid from dietary sources, and also made in the body from phenylalanine that the thyroid gland combines with iodine to make thyroid hormone

underactive thyroid—casual term for hypothyroidism; exists when the thyroid gland does not produce adequate thyroid hormone

Unithroid—brand of levothyroxine (synthetic T4 supplement)

Westhroid—brand of natural desiccated thyroid

Wilson's rT3 dominance syndrome—condition in which high levels of cortisol are believed to interfere with T4-to-T3 conversion, resulting in a high level of rT3; produces symptoms of hypothyroidism but with inconclusive blood-test results; usually treated with time-release T3 in a cycle of increasing and decreasing doses

yoga—Eastern system of body poses and meditation for physical conditioning and stress relief

Appendix

B

Additional Resources

In addition to these books, visit Dr. Rothfeld's Web site, *www.thyroidbalance.com*, which provides information about traditional and alternative thyroid medicine.

Aronson, Diane, and the staff of RESOLVE. *Resolving Infertility.* New York: Quill/HarperCollins, 1999.

Barnes, Broda, M.D., and Lawrence Galton. *Hypothyroidism: The Unsuspected Illness.* New York: Harper & Row, 1976.

Domar, Alice, Ph.D., and Henry Dreher. *Healing Mind, Healthy Woman.* New York: Dell Books, 1996.

Gastelu, Daniel. *The Complete Nutritional Supplements Buyer's Guide.* New York: Three Rivers Press, 2000.

Harbar, Sari, and Sara Altshul O'Donnell. *The Woman's Book of Healing Herbs.* Emmaus, PA: Rodale Press, Inc., 1999.

Hoffman, Eileen, M.D. *Our Health, Our Lives: A Revolutionary Approach to Total Health Care for Women.* New York: Pocket Books/Simon & Schuster, 1995.

McClain, Gary, Ph.D., and Eve Adamson, MFA. *The Complete Idiot's Guide to Zen Living.* Indianapolis: Alpha Books, 2001.

Moyers, Bill. *Healing and the Mind.* New York: Doubleday, 1993.

Northrup, Christiane, M.D. *Women's Bodies, Women's Wisdom: Creating Physical and Emotional Health and Healing.* New York: Bantam Books, 1998 (revised edition).

Reader's Digest Magic and Medicine of Plants. Pleasantville, NY: Reader's Digest Association, 1994.

Romaine, Deborah S., and Jennifer B. Marks, M.D. *Syndrome X: Managing Insulin Resistance* (with a foreword by Glenn S. Rothfeld, M.D.). New York: HarperCollins Publishers, 2000.

Rothfeld, Glenn S., M.D., M.Ac., and Suzanne LeVert. *Ginko Biloba: An Herbal Fountain of Youth for Your Brain.* New York: Dell Publishing, 1998.

Rothfeld, Glenn S., M.D., M.Ac., and Suzanne LeVert. *Folic Acid and the Amazing B Vitamins.* New York: Berkeley Publishing Group, 2000.

Rothfeld, Glenn S., M.D., M.Ac., and Suzanne LeVert. *The Acupuncture Response.* New York: Contemporary Books, 2002.

Rowe, John W., M.D., and Robert L. Kahn, Ph.D. *Successful Aging: The MacArthur Foundation Study.* New York: Pantheon Books, 1998.

Sivananda Yoga Center's *The Sivananda Companion to Yoga.* New York: Fireside/Simon & Schuster, 1983.

Index